SUZANNE BYRD

ADHD and Sex

A Woman's Perspective

First published by Mental Health Publishing 2025

Copyright © 2025 by Suzanne Byrd

All rights reserved. No part of this publication may be reproduced, stored or transmitted in any form or by any means, electronic, mechanical, photocopying, recording, scanning, or otherwise without written permission from the publisher. It is illegal to copy this book, post it to a website, or distribute it by any other means without permission.

First edition

This book was professionally typeset on Reedsy. Find out more at reedsy.com

Contents

1. Introduction – Why ADHD & Sex? — 1
2. Understanding ADHD in Women — 10
3. Female Sexuality & ADHD – Myths vs. Reality — 20
4. Self-Esteem, Body Image, and ADHD — 30
5. Intimacy, Connection, and Sensory Overload — 40
6. Communication in Relationships — 51
7. ADHD, Trauma, and Sexuality — 63
8. Medication, Libido, and Alternatives — 73
9. Empowerment and Self-Discovery — 85
10. Moving Forward – Embracing Complexity — 96

1

Introduction – Why ADHD & Sex?

Setting the Stage

It's early morning, and I'm already late—again. My car keys have somehow migrated to the bathroom counter, my favorite bra is missing in the laundry pile, and I'm juggling a half-eaten bagel while trying to respond to a text from my boss. My mind is racing through half a dozen unfinished tasks, and even though this whirlwind is my everyday reality, I often feel misunderstood.

For women living with Attention Deficit Hyperactivity Disorder (ADHD), life can sometimes feel like a constant struggle of too much stimulation but never enough organization. We shuttle between fleeting moments of hyperfocus and seemingly endless bouts of distraction. Some days, it's exhilarating. On others, it's exhausting. Yet, in the midst of this balancing act—amid busy schedules, medication management, and mindful routines—there is an aspect of life that often receives little attention: our sexual experiences.

Discussions about ADHD typically revolve around academic performance, employment struggles, or maintaining a household. Sexuality, on the other hand, is rarely at the forefront. For many women, talking openly about sex is already laden with cultural taboos and personal vulnerabilities. Add ADHD to that mix, and the conversation can become even more complex. This book, *ADHD & Sex: A Woman's Perspective*, aims to shine light on an overlooked yet profoundly impactful topic: how ADHD informs, shapes, and sometimes challenges our sexual identity, pleasure, and intimate relationships.

Understanding the Overlooked Intersection

When it comes to ADHD, doctors and mental health professionals have historically used diagnostic criteria based on studies of young boys. Over time, this skewed lens missed a huge swath of the female experience. Women often exhibit fewer overt hyperactive behaviors, tending to internalize symptoms or present with daydreaminess, anxiety, or depressive tendencies. This difference has contributed to later diagnoses or misdiagnoses. And while awareness is improving, there is still much to be done.

Sexuality, similarly, has its share of misunderstandings, misconceptions, and stigmatization—especially for women. We face cultural scripts about what "good" sexual behavior looks like. We're expected to strike a delicate balance between confidence and modesty, between being adventurous and not "too much." These complexities multiply for women with ADHD. Traits like impulsivity might influence our sexual decisions. Inattentiveness might make it hard to focus on pleasure. Hyperfocus can lead to periods of intense intimacy, but also swift drops in interest. Emotional dysregulation can create peaks of passion followed by valleys of shame or anxiety. And yet, these unique dimensions are rarely discussed openly.

What happens when ADHD meets sex? Let's consider a scenario: imagine a woman who experiences hyperfocus on a new romantic partner. During that initial honeymoon phase, the ADHD-driven fascination can be so intense that it almost feels like an obsession. Conversations last for hours, texts light up phones day and night, and sex can become an all-encompassing pastime. Then, a few months in, the "newness" wears off. ADHD's challenges with sustained attention might surface, leaving her partner confused or hurt as the intensity suddenly shifts. She might wonder if there's something wrong with her for not being able to maintain that level of interest. He or she might wonder why it feels as though a switch was flipped. Unaddressed, these issues can quickly spiral, breeding resentment or misunderstanding.

This book will show that these experiences aren't abnormalities or moral failings; they're part of a complex interplay of neurological wiring, environmental influences, and personal histories. By exploring these layers, we can begin to remove shame and replace it with informed choices, self-compassion, and constructive communication.

Goals for This Book

Our first goal here is **awareness**. Often, women with ADHD have never connected their symptoms to their sexual wellness or relationship satisfaction. By shining a spotlight on this often-neglected topic, we can foster a sense of recognition and relief— an "aha!" moment that confirms, "I'm not alone in feeling this way."

Next, we aim to provide **practical tools**. Knowledge is a powerful start, but putting that knowledge into practice is essential. Through real-life anecdotes, evidence-based research, and exercises, each chapter will delve into how ADHD influences self-esteem, body image, desire, orgasm, emotional intimacy, and relationship dynamics. We will look at medication's impact, suggest communication strategies, and discuss the interplay between ADHD and trauma.

Finally, we want to cultivate **community** and **self-compassion**. Dealing with the complexities of ADHD can feel isolating, and discussing sexual struggles can amplify that isolation. A core message throughout this book is that no woman with ADHD is alone. There is a community of others who face similar challenges, triumphs, and discoveries. By sharing stories, we can find solidarity and support.

Laying the Groundwork for a Holistic Perspective

You might wonder: Why focus on women specifically? Isn't ADHD & sex relevant to everyone? The short answer is yes—anyone with ADHD can be affected by it in their sex life. However, gender norms and hormonal fluctuations heavily shape women's experiences. For instance, the menstrual cycle can exacerbate or lessen ADHD symptoms. Hormonal birth control or menopause introduce yet another layer of potential influence. Culturally, women often grapple with contradictory messages about how to express—or repress—sexual desire. These factors collectively create a unique vantage point for women that deserves dedicated attention.

Additionally, women typically face higher rates of internalizing mental health issues, such as anxiety and depression, which can be intricately linked to self-esteem in the bedroom. The guilt or shame that often accompanies ADHD-related forgetfulness or impulsive behavior can easily spill over into sex. Perhaps you've forgotten an anniversary or missed your partner's signals for intimacy because you were hyperfocused on your phone or a project. These common ADHD occurrences can pile on negative self-talk, making you feel unworthy or incompetent. Addressing these underlying emotional challenges is crucial for fostering healthier sexual connections and personal fulfillment.

Embracing a Sex-Positive Framework

A foundational aspect of this book is a **sex-positive outlook**—a belief that consensual sexual exploration and expression is healthy, beneficial, and integral to personal well-being. For many women, ADHD might add spice, adventure, and spontaneity to their sex lives. For others, it can introduce anxiety or frustration. Regardless of how ADHD shows up, the aim is not to label any facet of sexual expression as inherently "good" or "bad." Instead, we aim to offer a deeper understanding of why certain patterns emerge and how to navigate them in ways that uplift and empower.

We'll discuss the importance of understanding **desire discrepancy**—the mismatch in libido that can occur between partners or even within oneself at different times. We'll explore **sensory sensitivities**, which can turn certain textures, scents, or touches from pleasurable to overwhelming in seconds. We'll also highlight the role of **emotional regulation**, noting how an ADHD brain's heightened reactivity can either fuel passion or ignite conflict. Each of these elements is crucial for a holistic understanding of ADHD-informed sexuality.

Normalizing the Conversation

One of the biggest barriers to knowledge is silence. Women are often socialized to keep sexual topics private, and ADHD symptoms—especially executive function challenges—can foster feelings of embarrassment. Admitting that you struggle with basic organizational tasks can be difficult enough; admitting that your ADHD affects your ability to orgasm, concentrate during sex, or handle relationship conflicts might feel even more daunting. Yet, speaking candidly is the first step toward education, validation, and problem-solving.

Throughout this book, you'll find interviews and anecdotes from women with ADHD who have navigated these waters. Hearing their stories can illuminate that the ups and downs you might face in your own life are not isolated incidents but part of a broader pattern shared by many. This normalization can dissolve shame, encouraging healthier ways to address challenges.

How to Use This Book

Each chapter is structured to build on the previous one, creating a comprehensive roadmap. Here's a quick overview of what you can expect:

1. **Foundations of ADHD in Women**: We'll delve deeper into the biological, psychological, and cultural factors that shape a woman's ADHD experience, laying the groundwork for all subsequent discussions.
2. **Myths vs. Realities** around ADHD and female sexuality, breaking down common misconceptions and illuminating

research findings.
3. **Self-Esteem and Body Image** in the context of ADHD, highlighting how negative self-talk or disordered thinking can impact sexual confidence.
4. **Intimacy and Sensory Overload**, exploring techniques for managing sensitivities and enhancing emotional closeness.
5. **Communication** strategies within relationships, focusing on how to share ADHD-related challenges with partners and how to work through conflicts.
6. **ADHD, Trauma, and Sexuality**, a nuanced look at how some women with ADHD may be more susceptible to certain traumatic experiences and how healing intersects with intimacy.
7. **Medication and Libido**, examining how different treatments for ADHD can affect sexual desire and function, plus alternatives to support overall sexual well-being.
8. **Empowerment and Self-Discovery**, providing exercises and reflections for understanding one's own desires, preferences, and needs.
9. **Moving Forward**, with an emphasis on long-term strategies, advocacy, and building supportive communities.

Feel free to read the chapters sequentially for a full understanding, or jump to the areas most relevant to you. Because ADHD can manifest differently for each person, not all advice will apply equally. Use this book as a resource and springboard for your own explorations, taking what resonates and leaving the rest.

Looking Ahead

If you've picked up this book, it's likely because you're ready to gain insights into your own life or to better support someone you love. Maybe you've had an inkling that ADHD influences your sexual relationships, or perhaps you're searching for ways to communicate your needs to a partner. Whatever brings you here, know that this journey is about embracing complexity. ADHD is multifaceted, touching every aspect of life—from how we manage our time to how we experience joy, pleasure, and connection in the bedroom.

Understanding the interplay between ADHD and sexuality isn't just about tackling problems; it's also about discovering new avenues for pleasure, closeness, and self-expression. Many women find that once they become aware of the ways ADHD impacts their sex life, they can channel the best parts of their neurology—like creativity, spontaneity, and heightened sensitivity—to enhance their experiences. This process isn't about eradicating ADHD-related traits but learning to harness them effectively.

An Invitation

I invite you to approach the following chapters with curiosity and compassion. You may find some sections resonate immediately, while others prompt deeper self-reflection over time. Keep a journal or notes if you can, jotting down thoughts, feelings, or questions that arise. Consider sharing your reflections with a trusted friend, a therapist, or a partner. By bringing these insights into conversations, you'll help dismantle the stigma around ADHD and sexuality, both for yourself and for the broader community of women who share these experiences.

As we begin this journey together, remember that every story is unique. Your challenges, desires, fears, and triumphs may look different from another woman's, and that's okay. The goal is not to fit a standard mold but to discover your personal strategies for leading a fulfilling and empowered sexual life. Let's step forward with an open mind, ready to learn and unlearn, to embrace and evolve.

In the next chapter, we'll deepen our exploration of ADHD in women. We'll discuss the nuances of how ADHD presents differently from the male-dominated diagnostic model, the hormonal ebbs and flows that exacerbate or soothe symptoms, and the ways in which these facets inevitably impact our sexual identities. By the end of Chapter Two, you'll have a clearer blueprint of your ADHD landscape—one that can help you make better sense of the sexual challenges or strengths you've encountered.

Thank you for starting this journey. Whether you're newly diagnosed or have known about your ADHD for years, whether you're single or partnered, queer or straight, in your twenties or in your sixties—this book is for you. Let's dive in.

2

Understanding ADHD in Women

The Bigger Picture

When physicians and researchers first started studying Attention Deficit Hyperactivity Disorder (ADHD), their focus often skewed toward hyperactive young boys who struggled to sit still in classroom settings. Over the decades, this led to diagnostic criteria that largely reflected a "male" presentation of the disorder—emphasizing external behaviors like impulsivity and restlessness. For many years, society believed these boys would simply "grow out of it," ignoring the reality that ADHD is a lifelong neurological condition. Meanwhile, the ADHD experiences of girls and women often flew under the radar, largely because their symptoms could manifest differently or be more easily masked.

In recent years, however, a growing body of research has begun to illuminate a more nuanced picture. We now know that ADHD is not a childhood disorder—nor is it limited to males. It affects people of all genders, persisting into adulthood, and it can show up in a variety of ways that defy the early stereotypes. By diving into these nuances—particularly around the female experience—we gain a clearer understanding of how ADHD shapes identity, self-esteem, and yes, sexuality.

The Core Components of ADHD

Before we zero in on gender-specific variations, it's helpful to review the key features of ADHD. Typically, ADHD is characterized by one or more of the following symptom clusters:

1. **Inattention**: Difficulty focusing, sustaining attention over longer tasks, forgetfulness, disorganization, and frequent distractibility.
2. **Hyperactivity**: An inner sense of restlessness, fidgeting, difficulty engaging in quiet activities, and a need for constant movement.
3. **Impulsivity**: Acting on urges or making decisions hastily, interrupting conversations, or engaging in risky behaviors without fully considering consequences.

Diagnostically, these clusters often manifest in three types of ADHD:

- **Predominantly Inattentive Type**
- **Predominantly Hyperactive-Impulsive Type**
- **Combined Type** (a mix of inattentive and hyperactive-impulsive symptoms)

In reality, however, ADHD symptoms exist on a spectrum. Two individuals with the same "type" might still experience daily life very differently. This diversity of presentation is especially evident when we examine how ADHD shows up in women.

The Unique Female Presentation

For many women, ADHD symptoms can be more subtle or internalized compared to the proverbial hyperactive boy running laps around a classroom. Instead of boundless external energy, a woman with ADHD might be daydreamy or quietly disorganized—often described in her youth as "the spacey girl" who gazed out the window during class. Alternatively, if she does exhibit hyperactivity, it might manifest as constant fidgeting, leg shaking, or racing thoughts rather than overtly disruptive behaviors.

This distinction matters because quieter, more inattentive presentations are frequently overlooked by teachers, parents, and even medical professionals. As a result, many women do not receive an ADHD diagnosis until later in life—sometimes in their thirties, forties, or beyond. For these women, realizing they have ADHD can be both a revelation and a relief, explaining a lifetime of feeling different, scattered, or perpetually behind.

Emotional Regulation and Masking

Another key factor in female ADHD is emotional regulation. While difficulties with impulsivity and emotional control are often noted in men and boys, women may channel these challenges inward. They may become skilled at "masking"—that is, consciously or unconsciously hiding their symptoms to meet societal expectations of politeness, calmness, and capability. Over time, this masking can lead to chronic stress, burnout, and internalized shame. It's not uncommon for women with ADHD to develop anxiety or depressive disorders, in part because constantly pretending everything is fine becomes exhausting.

Masking can also play out in social and romantic contexts. A woman might appear put-together on the surface, yet behind closed doors, she struggles to manage everyday tasks or maintain her sense of self-worth. The pressure to be a "good partner" or a "perfect mom" can heighten these feelings. When her sex life comes into the picture, it may become just one more area where she worries she's falling short or not meeting expectations—an anxiety that can dampen desire and sexual satisfaction.

Hormonal Influences

In addition to cultural factors, female biology adds another layer of complexity. Hormones—particularly estrogen—can directly affect neurotransmitters in the brain such as dopamine and serotonin, which play critical roles in ADHD. Women often notice that their ADHD symptoms fluctuate across different life stages:

Menstrual Cycle

- Estrogen levels rise and fall during the menstrual cycle. Some women experience sharper ADHD symptoms in the days leading up to their period (when estrogen dips), reporting higher irritability, decreased concentration, and a reduced libido.

Pregnancy and Postpartum

- Pregnancy brings massive hormonal shifts. Some women with ADHD find relief from certain symptoms during pregnancy, while others feel more disorganized and anxious. After childbirth, the sudden drop in estrogen can exacerbate both ADHD and postpartum mood issues.

Perimenopause and Menopause

- As estrogen gradually declines, some women experience a noticeable intensification of ADHD symptoms. This change can coincide with hot flashes, sleep disturbances, and mood swings, creating a perfect storm of factors impacting sexual desire and comfort.

These hormonal fluctuations underscore the importance of adopting a dynamic approach to ADHD management. Strategies that work effectively during one phase might need recalibration in another. Understanding these shifts can help women navigate their changing libidos, energy levels, and emotional states, ultimately enabling them to communicate more clearly with partners about what they need—both in and out of the bedroom.

Impact on Daily Life and Self-Esteem

We often hear about ADHD's impact on tasks like time management or organization, but less attention is paid to its effect on how women see themselves. When every day brings reminders that you're "failing" at basic adulting—missing deadlines, misplacing keys, forgetting appointments—it can take a toll on self-esteem. Add to that the cultural expectations placed upon women (to be nurturing, responsible, and orderly), and it's easy to see why many internalize the idea that they're somehow flawed or incompetent.

This negative self-perception can bleed into one's sexual identity. Feeling incompetent or scattered during the day makes it hard to shift into a confident, empowered mindset at night. A woman with ADHD might worry about being "too much" or "not enough" in bed, second-guessing her desires or performance. Alternatively, she might engage in impulsive sexual behavior to seek validation, only to feel guilt or confusion afterwards.

The ADHD Mind and Desire

On a more hopeful note, ADHD also brings traits that can enhance intimacy. For example, the capacity for **hyperfocus** can be a superpower in the right context. During the early stages of a romance, hyperfocus can create an intense bond. You might become thoroughly enthralled with a partner, noticing every detail, sharing long conversations, and experiencing heightened sexual excitement. Many women with ADHD describe this period as exhilarating, yet it can fade just as rapidly when novelty wears off or responsibilities demand attention elsewhere.

Additionally, the **adventurous spirit** often seen in ADHD—rooted in a constant search for novelty and stimulation—can lead to imaginative sex, playful experimentation, and a willingness to explore uncharted territories of pleasure. This openness can enrich relationships, provided there is mutual respect and communication.

Still, balancing these strengths with the challenges can be tricky. If hyperfocus wanes or restlessness takes over, a once-passionate relationship may stagnate. If emotional dysregulation flares up, conflicts can escalate quickly. Recognizing these patterns helps illuminate why some relationships burn bright and fast, while others never fully ignite.

Comorbidities: Anxiety and Depression

Many women with ADHD also grapple with anxiety and depression—sometimes as direct consequences of years spent feeling misunderstood, overwhelmed, or inadequate. These co-occurring conditions can further complicate sexual relationships. Anxiety might lead to excessive worries about performance, rejection, or intimacy itself. Depression can lower libido and foster disconnection from one's body, dampening sexual pleasure.

Medical and therapeutic interventions can be crucial here. Some women find relief in medication that targets both ADHD and mood disorders, while others benefit from therapy modalities like Cognitive Behavioral Therapy (CBT) or Dialectical Behavior Therapy (DBT). Creating a holistic plan that addresses ADHD's interplay with mental health is fundamental for nurturing both general well-being and sexual vitality.

ADHD in Different Relationship Dynamics

Another critical layer is how ADHD manifests within diverse relationship structures:

- **Long-Term Partnerships**: Over time, ADHD patterns can lead to a "caretaker" dynamic if the non-ADHD partner takes on more tasks, leading to resentment or an uneven emotional workload.
- **Casual Dating**: Women who date casually might rely on

impulsivity or novelty-seeking to spark interest. That can be fun initially but may lead to inconsistent or unstable connections if ADHD-related communication challenges arise.
- **Polyamory or Non-Monogamy**: Multiple relationships can provide more novelty and variety, which some women with ADHD find appealing. However, maintaining organization, communication, and emotional balance across several partners can be especially taxing.
- **Same-Sex Relationships**: While the dynamic may differ from heterosexual norms, the underlying ADHD traits—such as impulsivity or inattentiveness—remain the same, requiring similar navigation and communication.

Regardless of the relationship format, understanding your own ADHD patterns—when you're likely to thrive, when you need extra support, and when you might be more susceptible to conflict—can help you build healthier, more satisfying connections.

A Crucial Foundation for Sexual Exploration

Why does all of this matter for sex specifically? Because sexuality doesn't exist in a vacuum. Your beliefs about yourself, your body, and your worthiness of pleasure are deeply influenced by how you operate in the broader world. If you've spent decades grappling with internalized shame or anxiety, you may struggle to express your sexual needs confidently. If you rely on impulsivity for excitement, you could find it challenging to slow down and savor intimacy with a long-term partner.

Conversely, when you harness the positive aspects of ADHD—

creativity, curiosity, spontaneity—you can unlock new dimensions of sexual exploration. Recognizing your triggers and tendencies also equips you to communicate your desires and boundaries more effectively. This form of self-awareness is essential; it's the bedrock upon which you can build a fulfilling, dynamic, and, yes, even adventurous sex life.

Looking Forward: Bridging Understanding into Action

Now that we've established the basics of how ADHD often differs for women, the next step is to apply this understanding to our everyday experiences and intimate lives. If you relate to any of the descriptions above—late diagnosis, struggles with self-esteem, fluctuating symptoms, or emotional highs and lows—know that you're not alone. Countless women share this journey, and many have found ways to thrive by learning to work with, rather than against, their ADHD.

In the coming chapters, we'll delve deeper into specific areas—like self-esteem, body image, and communication strategies—that can directly impact sexual satisfaction. We'll also discuss how to handle sensory sensitivities and emotional dysregulation during intimacy. You'll gain concrete tools, from journaling prompts to conversation starters, designed to help you translate abstract knowledge into practical changes.

This process of understanding is not a one-time task; it's a continuous evolution. ADHD is dynamic, and your needs may shift over time or under stress. Embracing that evolution—staying curious about your body, your mind, and your relationships—can lead to a more nuanced, compassionate, and ultimately more satisfying approach to sex.

Final Thoughts

Understanding ADHD in women is about more than just diagnosis. It's about recognizing how neurological wiring, societal pressures, and personal experiences intersect to shape everything—from your daily routines to your deepest desires. For too long, women have navigated these challenges in silence, uncertain whether their struggles or sudden shifts in libido were "normal." By shedding light on this topic, we validate the countless women who have felt sidelined or misunderstood.

In the next chapter, we'll further expand on how cultural myths and stereotypes warp our views of women with ADHD—particularly in the realm of sexuality. We'll dissect the narratives that label ADHD women as either disinterested in sex or hypersexual, showing how these oversimplifications can obscure the real complexities. We'll also begin exploring evidence-based research to help ground our discussions in science as well as personal testimony.

As you proceed, take a moment to reflect on your own experiences. Which parts of ADHD resonate most for you? Have hormonal shifts affected your sense of well-being or your sexual interest? Do you notice patterns of masking or impulsivity in your relationships? Identifying these elements early on will help you adapt the insights and strategies offered throughout this book, ensuring they speak directly to your reality.

You deserve a fulfilling, autonomous, and joyful relationship with both your ADHD and your sexuality. And that journey begins with understanding—understanding that every challenge can also be an invitation to grow, to innovate, and to build a life that respects and even celebrates the complexities of the ADHD mind.

3

Female Sexuality & ADHD – Myths vs. Reality

Stereotypes and Stigma

From the moment we first hear about ADHD, many of us internalize a familiar set of clichés: it's the young boy who can't sit still in school, or the teenager impulsively blurting answers in class. These stereotypes often leave out the experiences of women, especially in the realm of sexuality. When it comes to intimate life, two particular tropes seem to surface repeatedly:

- **Women with ADHD are disinterested or "frigid."**

Here, ADHD-related inattentiveness or executive function challenges may be interpreted as sexual indifference. If a woman struggles to maintain focus in the bedroom, or if her attraction to a partner waxes and wanes, people sometimes assume she simply doesn't like sex.

- **Women with ADHD are hypersexual or "too much."**

On the flip side, another pervasive myth casts women with ADHD as wild, impulsive, and unable to control their sexual urges. The same restlessness or novelty-seeking that drives ADHD can be twisted into a caricature of licentious behavior.

Neither stereotype paints a fair picture. Instead, they oversimplify a complex interplay of traits—like impulsivity, hyperfocus, emotional regulation, and fluctuating libido—into a binary. These labels also carry moral judgment that can shame or confuse women who don't fit neatly into either category. The stigma is compounded by the fact that female sexuality is already policed by cultural expectations. Women are supposed to be "just right": not too eager, not too detached, not too vocal, not too silent. Add ADHD to the equation, and the pressure can feel overwhelming.

The Myth of Disinterest

Why does the myth of disinterest persist? One factor is that ADHD, particularly the inattentive subtype, can manifest as daydreaming or difficulty staying present. If a woman's mind wanders during sexual intimacy, her partner might interpret that as boredom or lack of attraction. In reality, her mind could simply be racing with unrelated thoughts—unfinished tasks, emotional worries, or random curiosities. This mental chatter doesn't necessarily reflect a lack of desire; it's a byproduct of her neurological wiring.

Moreover, executive function deficits can influence a woman's ability to plan for or engage in sexual encounters. Scheduling a date night or setting aside time for intimacy might require organizational skills that are harder for her to maintain. She might also struggle with transitions, such as switching from "work mode" or "mom mode" to "romantic partner mode." These difficulties can inadvertently lower the frequency of sexual activity, which may be misconstrued as disinterest. In truth, the woman might crave more intimacy but feels hampered by the practical and mental barriers that ADHD imposes.

Another dimension to consider is **rejection sensitivity**, a trait commonly reported by people with ADHD. This heightened sensitivity can make the fear of rejection—even a minor one—loom large, leading some women to avoid initiating sex. They don't want to risk a "not tonight" response that could confirm their worst anxieties about being unwanted or undesirable. Over time, this avoidance can morph into a self-fulfilling prophecy, where lack of sexual engagement becomes a pattern. From the outside, it may look like disinterest. On the inside, it's often rooted in fear, overwhelm, or a web of logistical challenges.

The Myth of Hypersexuality

On the other end of the spectrum, some people assume that ADHD's impulsivity translates to promiscuity or hypersexual behavior. It's true that impulsivity can drive some women with ADHD to seek sexual experiences more spontaneously, driven by the moment's excitement. Hyperfocus can also supercharge romantic or sexual pursuits during the early stages of attraction, creating an intense bond. But labeling women as purely "hypersexual" flattens this complexity into a one-note caricature.

First, not all impulsive decisions are rooted in a craving for sex alone; sometimes, it's the allure of novelty or the desire for connection that pushes a woman to dive into an encounter. In some instances, this can lead to regrets or emotional fallout if the situation didn't align with her deeper values or needs. Rather than a "wild streak," this might be a result of difficulty in self-regulation—trouble pausing to consider long-term implications during moments of high excitement.

Furthermore, a woman might exhibit periods of increased sexual interest and then experience abrupt drops in libido. This fluctuation can stem from ADHD's cyclical nature, hormonal changes, or shifting external stressors. Mistaking a temporary spike in sexual energy for a permanent state of hypersexuality disregards how fluid desire can be for anyone—especially those grappling with ADHD's emotional and attentional swings.

The Nuances of Desire

In reality, most women with ADHD exist on a broad, ever-shifting continuum of sexual desire. Some may consistently lean toward high libido, others might lean toward low, and many fluctuate somewhere in between depending on factors like:

- **Stress Levels**: Anxiety and overload at work or home can stifle libido.
- **Medication**: Stimulants can sometimes dampen or heighten sexual desire, depending on the individual. Antidepressants used for comorbid anxiety or depression also affect libido.
- **Relationship Quality**: Emotional closeness, intimacy, and sense of security can make or break one's interest in sex.
- **Hormonal Cycle**: A woman may feel particularly responsive around ovulation and less so during PMS or menopause.

Desire itself is a complex interplay of psychological, emotional, and physical elements. ADHD adds another layer to this mix by influencing how a woman processes stimuli, regulates emotions, and manages energy. The important takeaway is that there isn't a single "normal" trajectory of desire for women with ADHD. Each individual's patterns can look different—and can change over time.

Cultural Scripts and Sexuality

The cultural scripts that dictate how women "should" behave can also intensify confusion for those with ADHD. Women are told to be polite, nurturing, and organized—traits that may clash with ADHD symptoms like forgetfulness, impulsivity, or disorganization. When it comes to sexuality, societal expectations pile on further: be alluring, but not "easy"; be adventurous, but not "kinky"; be confident, but not "overbearing."

For a woman who is already grappling with the daily friction of ADHD, these contradictory mandates can feel almost impossible to meet. She may find herself caught between wanting to express her authentic sexual desires and fearing how she'll be perceived. In some cases, she might swing between extremes—overcompensating in one area, then retreating in another—trying to find a balance that feels safe. Ironically, the pursuit of an "acceptable" sexual persona can disconnect her from the genuine exploration of what she actually wants or needs.

Fact-Checking with Research

While research on ADHD and female sexuality remains limited compared to broader studies on ADHD, a growing number of inquiries are shining light on these topics. Surveys and clinical observations indicate that many women with ADHD report **higher rates of sexual dissatisfaction** than their neurotypical peers. The reasons range from difficulty staying focused during intimate moments to emotional dysregulation that leads to conflicts with partners.

At the same time, there are also studies suggesting that women with ADHD can experience **richer sexual satisfaction** when their symptoms are well-managed, due to enhanced creativity, openness to novelty, and an intense capacity for connection during periods of hyperfocus. This apparent contradiction underscores the importance of individualized approaches rather than blanket assumptions. ADHD can be both an obstacle and an asset in the realm of sexuality, depending on context and coping strategies.

Additional research points to **co-occurring conditions** like anxiety, depression, or post-traumatic stress disorder (PTSD) as major influences on sexual health. Women with ADHD are at greater risk for these conditions, which can obscure the direct link between ADHD and sexual well-being. Unraveling what part of a woman's sexual challenges stem from ADHD and what part stem from broader mental health issues can be complex. Yet, doing so paves the way for targeted interventions and greater self-understanding.

Toward a Fuller Reality

What does the "real" experience of female sexuality and ADHD look like, beyond myths and stereotypes? While every woman's story will differ, a few common threads emerge:

1. **Fluidity of Interest**: Sexual desire can wax and wane, influenced by hormone levels, relationship contexts, and ADHD symptom management.
2. **High Sensitivity**: Emotional sensitivity can heighten both pleasure and pain, making intimacy deeply fulfilling at times and overwhelming at others.
3. **Complex Self-Expression**: Women with ADHD often have to navigate a maze of cultural expectations, personal preferences, and ADHD traits to define their unique style of sexual expression.
4. **Navigational Strategies**: Practical tools—such as scheduling intimate time, using mindfulness techniques to stay present, or consciously managing environment and sensory inputs—can shift the sexual experience from chaotic to pleasurable.

Rather than defaulting to reductive labels, we can embrace the reality that female sexuality under ADHD is just as varied, messy, and beautiful as any other sexual identity. The difference lies in the unique challenges and opportunities ADHD presents—challenges that can be mitigated with support, and opportunities that can enrich a woman's life in unexpected ways.

Shattering the Myths

One of the most empowering steps toward sexual fulfillment is **shattering the myths** that have silenced or stigmatized women with ADHD. Recognizing that neither "frigid" nor "hypersexual" are valid descriptors for most women with ADHD frees them to explore their sexuality without shame or confusion. It also opens the door to honest communication with partners, friends, and medical professionals, who can offer more targeted and compassionate support.

If you've ever found yourself pigeonholed by these myths—whether from external sources or your own internal self-talk—know that you have the power to reject them. Your sexual identity is not a fixed label but a dynamic, evolving facet of who you are. Yes, ADHD will influence how you experience sex, but it does not define your worth or your capacity for intimacy. Challenging these stereotypes is part of breaking down broader societal stigma around mental health and sexuality, and your voice in that conversation is invaluable.

Looking Ahead: A Path Forward

Understanding these myths is the first step in transcending them. The next chapters will delve into more specific areas that shape your lived sexual experience, including self-esteem, body image, emotional regulation, and communication in relationships. We'll discuss practical techniques to manage overstimulation, ways to harness hyperfocus for greater pleasure, and strategies to mitigate impulsivity when it proves more harmful than helpful.

Before moving on, take a moment to reflect on the stories

or stereotypes you've encountered about women with ADHD—stories that might have shaped your perception of your own sexuality. What threads feel accurate? Which feel misplaced or harmful? By identifying these influences, you can start replacing them with more nuanced insights, ones that honor the complexity of your experiences rather than reduce them to a single narrative.

Remember, your sexuality is an extension of your overall well-being. As you learn more about ADHD and discover tools that support your unique wiring, you'll also gain insights that can enrich your sexual life. Whether you view sex as a playful exploration, a spiritual connection, or a source of deep emotional bonding—understanding how ADHD factors in can make the journey smoother, more self-compassionate, and deeply fulfilling.

Conclusion

The third chapter of our exploration has peeled back the layers of myths surrounding female sexuality and ADHD. Far from being a tidy issue of "too little" or "too much" desire, the reality lies in a vibrant spectrum shaped by neurology, hormones, personal history, and social context. As we continue, we'll build on this foundation to address challenges like body image, self-esteem, and communication—elements that powerfully intersect with ADHD to influence a woman's intimate life.

Next, we turn our focus to **Chapter Four: Self-Esteem, Body Image, and ADHD**. Here, we'll explore how negative self-talk and disordered thinking around body image can intersect with ADHD's emotional ups and downs. By understanding these patterns, you'll be better equipped to foster a kinder, more confident relationship with yourself—one that naturally extends into sexual self-expression.

Remember, breaking down these myths is an ongoing process. Each time you name and challenge a stereotype, you free up more space to define your sexuality on your own terms—an essential step in reclaiming agency and finding fulfillment in every aspect of your life.

4

Self-Esteem, Body Image, and ADHD

The Power of Self-Perception

Self-esteem shapes the lens through which we experience the world. It influences our decision-making, our relationships, and even our willingness to explore and enjoy our own bodies. When a woman has ADHD, the interplay between her neurology and her sense of self can become particularly complex. Tasks that seem effortless for others—like arriving on time, completing errands without mishap, or remembering important dates—may require Herculean energy. The repeated feeling of "failing" at everyday life can sow seeds of self-doubt. Over time, this doubt can infiltrate how she views her body, her attractiveness, and her worthiness of love and pleasure.

For many women with ADHD, the process of building—or rebuilding—self-esteem includes unlearning the idea that they are inherently "flawed." Learning to see ADHD traits as differences rather than deficits can be transformative. Yet, even armed with a new perspective, deeply ingrained narratives

Linking ADHD Traits to Negative Self-Talk

ADHD affects not just how a woman thinks but also how she talks to herself. Throughout childhood and adolescence, a girl with undiagnosed or misunderstood ADHD may hear criticisms from teachers, relatives, or peers. She might be labeled "lazy" because she struggles with organization, or "careless" because she misplaces important items. These external judgments often mutate into an internal monologue that says, "I'm never good enough," or, "I can't do anything right."

Negative self-talk can take on a life of its own in adulthood, particularly around body image. For instance, a woman might start to blame her body for her ADHD symptoms: "If only I looked a certain way, maybe I'd be taken more seriously," or "I should be more disciplined, but I'm not—this must mean I'm unworthy." This spiral of thought can be amplified by the fact that ADHD can complicate self-care routines such as regular exercise, balanced eating, or consistent sleep schedules.

Emotional dysregulation adds another layer. Many women with ADHD experience intense emotional highs and lows. When self-esteem is low, a passing comment about weight or appearance can feel devastating, reinforcing a belief of unworthiness. Conversely, even a small compliment can spark euphoric confidence—until the next self-doubt creeps in. It's a rollercoaster that can make body acceptance feel like a moving target.

Cultural and Social Influences

We can't discuss body image without acknowledging the cultural messages bombarding women every day. Magazine covers, social media feeds, and celebrity culture often peddle an idealized version of femininity—thin yet curvy, perpetually youthful, and effortlessly stylish. For women with ADHD, maintaining that polished facade can be challenging. Executive functioning issues might make it tough to keep up with elaborate beauty routines or consistently plan nutritious meals. Sensory sensitivities could mean certain fabrics or clothing styles are physically uncomfortable, limiting wardrobe choices.

Moreover, women are socially conditioned to be "pleasing" in their appearance. Failing to align with these expectations can lead to additional shame or a sense of isolation. If a woman with ADHD repeatedly feels like she's falling short in other areas of life (work, academics, home management), the cultural pressure to also present a flawless body or stylish wardrobe can be overwhelming. This pressure can contribute to distorted self-perception and, in some cases, lead to disordered eating or exercise patterns.

Comparisons on social media further amplify the struggle. Scrolling through curated photos of friends or influencers who appear to have their lives together can spark negative self-comparisons: "Why can't I be that organized?" or "She has kids and still looks perfect; what's wrong with me?" When ADHD-driven disorganization intersects with a culture of visual perfection, it's a recipe for heightened self-criticism.

Body Image in ADHD

Body image isn't limited to weight or shape. It encompasses how a woman feels in her body—her sense of comfort, ownership, and connection to it. ADHD can shape that sense of connection in multiple ways:

1. **Mind-Body Disconnect**
2. Some women with ADHD experience a disconnect between mind and body, partly due to persistent mental chatter or distractibility. It can be hard to tune into physical cues—hunger, fullness, sexual arousal—when the brain is racing with unrelated thoughts.
3. **Sensory Sensitivities**
4. Heightened sensitivity to textures or pain can affect how a woman perceives her own body. She might feel easily irritated by certain clothing or dread intimate touch that feels uncomfortable. This can create an adversarial relationship with her body if she interprets these sensitivities as personal failings.
5. **Impulsive Eating or Restrictive Patterns**
6. ADHD's impulsivity can lead to binge eating or spur-of-the-moment dietary choices, while hyperfocus periods might cause a woman to forget to eat. Either extreme can fuel shame and contribute to a negative body image. Conversely, perfectionist tendencies—common in women who mask ADHD—may lead to rigid or restrictive eating as a means of control.
7. **Hormonal Fluctuations**
8. As discussed in earlier chapters, shifting hormone levels can intensify ADHD symptoms. A woman might notice

bloating, mood swings, or increased body awareness during certain parts of her cycle. If these changes coincide with heightened distractibility or irritability, the result can be a spike in body dissatisfaction.

Emotional Regulation and Body Acceptance

Despite the challenges, many women with ADHD develop deep wells of **resilience** and **compassion**—qualities that can be powerful tools in building healthier body image. Emotional regulation skills often need to be learned or consciously practiced, but once a woman begins to master them, she can apply those skills to self-talk about her body.

- **Identifying Emotional Triggers**: Because ADHD can involve swift emotional shifts, awareness is crucial. Does a certain type of social media post trigger self-criticism? Does a busy morning with multiple mishaps set the stage for negative body talk? By pinpointing triggers, it becomes easier to step back and reframe thought patterns before they spiral.
- **Mindful Pausing**: The classic ADHD trait of impulsivity can lead to quick judgments about body image—"I look terrible," "I hate how I feel today." Practicing a brief pause before allowing those thoughts to take over can create room for a more balanced perspective.
- **Self-Soothing Tactics**: Sometimes, no amount of rational thought will stop an emotional flood. In those moments, engaging the senses can help: taking a warm bath, lighting a favorite candle, or playing calming music. These strategies ground the body in a calmer state, making it easier to think kindly about oneself.

Fostering Self-Compassion

At its core, self-compassion is about treating yourself with the same kindness and understanding you'd offer a friend. This attitude is especially important for women with ADHD, who may have grown accustomed to negative feedback from both external sources and their internal dialogues. Strategies for nurturing self-compassion include:

1. **Reframing Mistakes**
2. If you skip a workout or have a disorganized day, remind yourself that setbacks are part of the human experience. A missed appointment or a binge-eating episode doesn't define your worth. With ADHD, mistakes are learning opportunities, not moral failings.
3. **Developing Body-Neutral Language**
4. For some, transitioning directly to body positivity can feel daunting. Body neutrality offers a gentler step: recognizing that your body is a vessel that enables you to live life, without placing judgment on whether it's "good" or "bad." Over time, this neutral stance can ease into genuine appreciation.
5. **Celebrating Non-Physical Traits**
6. Our culture often values appearance over other qualities, but focusing on your abilities—creativity, empathy, problem-solving—reminds you that beauty is only one dimension of who you are. ADHD often comes with strengths like adaptability or out-of-the-box thinking, qualities worth celebrating.
7. **Therapy and Support Groups**
8. Sometimes, the path to self-compassion requires outside

help. Therapies like Cognitive Behavioral Therapy (CBT) or Acceptance and Commitment Therapy (ACT) offer structured ways to challenge negative beliefs. Support groups—online or in-person—can also provide camaraderie and shared coping strategies.

From Body Image to Sexual Self-Confidence

A healthy, compassionate relationship with your body is the foundation for a satisfying sex life. If you're constantly battling self-doubt or berating yourself for perceived flaws, it's challenging to fully relax into pleasure. For women with ADHD, the journey to sexual self-confidence often begins with **body acceptance**—embracing the uniqueness of your form, your rhythms, and your sensory preferences.

- **Heightened Pleasure Through Mindfulness**: ADHD can derail focus, but mindfulness practices specifically tailored for sex—like paying attention to the sensation of touch, breath, or your partner's presence—can help anchor you in the moment. As you develop mindfulness in everyday life, you can bring that skill into intimate settings to counter negative self-talk about your body.
- **Communication About Sensitivities**: Open conversations with a partner about your sensory needs—whether you dislike certain textures or prefer a softer touch—can help prevent shame or discomfort. Feeling understood and respected in your body fosters greater self-esteem.
- **Celebrating Small Wins**: If you've had a lifetime of body-based insecurity, any step toward acceptance is significant. Did you try a new style of clothing that honors your sensory

comfort? Did you engage in an intimate encounter where you voiced your needs without self-judgment? These small victories build momentum, gradually rewiring how you see yourself.

Overcoming the Comparison Trap

Even as you work on self-esteem, it's crucial to remain vigilant about the **comparison trap**. Social media, pop culture, and even well-intentioned friends can unwittingly feed into damaging body ideals. For women with ADHD—who might already be grappling with emotional dysregulation—these comparisons can escalate quickly. Here are a few strategies to counteract them:

- **Curate Your Feed**: Unfollow accounts that make you feel worse about your body. Seek out body-positive or body-neutral influencers, ADHD advocates, and mental health professionals who provide uplifting, realistic content.
- **Remember the Highlight Reel**: Most people post their best moments online. The "perfect body" or "perfect life" you see is typically a carefully edited snapshot, not a full reality.
- **Stay Grounded in Personal Progress**: It can help to keep a journal where you track changes in your self-esteem or body image over time. Instead of comparing yourself to others, compare your present self to the past version of you who felt less confident.

Bridging Body Acceptance and Broader Well-Being

The positive shift in body image doesn't just improve sex—it radiates outward into all aspects of life. When you're less burdened by shame, you can more freely engage with hobbies, social events, or professional opportunities. You're also more likely to seek out health-related practices that suit you, whether it's a form of movement that feels joyful, a supportive diet that honors your body's needs, or a mindful relaxation technique that combats stress.

This holistic approach is especially beneficial for women with ADHD, whose day-to-day challenges can feel compartmentalized or scattered. By recognizing that body acceptance is intrinsically linked to emotional regulation, executive functioning, and interpersonal relationships, you can create a cohesive self-care plan. Rather than treating body image as an isolated issue, it becomes one piece of a well-rounded strategy for managing ADHD in a self-compassionate way.

Looking Forward

As you continue on this path of improving self-esteem and body image, remember that **progress is rarely linear**. You'll likely have good days when you feel confident and aligned, and others when negative thoughts resurface. These fluctuations are normal, especially when ADHD symptoms are at play. The key is to practice self-forgiveness for any perceived missteps and to celebrate each step forward, no matter how small.

In the next chapter, we'll delve into **Intimacy, Connection, and Sensory Overload**, examining how ADHD can shape everything from the desire for novelty to potential struggles with physical touch. Understanding how self-esteem intersects with these sensory experiences will be crucial. As you begin to heal your relationship with your body, you'll find it easier to communicate your needs, establish boundaries, and ultimately experience deeper pleasure and connection with yourself and others.

For now, take a moment to reflect. Notice how you feel in your body—perhaps there's tension in your shoulders or a flutter in your stomach. Can you approach those sensations with curiosity instead of judgment? If you catch yourself spiraling into negative self-talk, try pausing to breathe slowly and intentionally. Each small act of self-care is an investment in the relationship you have with the person who knows you best: yourself.

5

Intimacy, Connection, and Sensory Overload

The Layers of Intimacy

Picture this: you've finally found a quiet evening to spend with your partner. The candles are lit, the lights are low, and you've set aside your mental to-do list—at least for a moment. But just as you begin to relax into each other's arms, something disrupts the mood. Perhaps it's the faint hum of the air conditioner that you suddenly can't ignore, or the texture of your partner's shirt that feels oddly abrasive. In a flash, your sensory discomfort overshadows everything else. This sort of scenario is familiar for many women with ADHD, who often juggle heightened sensitivities alongside an active, sometimes restless mind.

But intimacy is more than just physical closeness. It's also the emotional tapestry that binds two people: trust, understanding, vulnerability, and open communication. Women with ADHD may face distinct hurdles on both fronts—navigating sensory sensitivities in the bedroom and managing the emotional complexities that shape genuine connection. These layers of intimacy can feel tangled, yet they also present opportunities for deeper understanding, creativity, and growth.

Understanding the ADHD Sensory Experience

ADHD isn't just about attention or impulsivity; it also frequently involves atypical sensory processing. Some individuals experience **hypersensitivity**, meaning certain stimuli—touch, smells, tastes, sounds—can feel unbearably intense. Others might contend with **hyposensitivity**, where sensory input doesn't register as strongly, leading to a craving for more stimulation or pressure. Many women oscillate between these two extremes, depending on stress levels, hormonal fluctuations, or simply the day's events.

During intimate moments, these sensory sensitivities can become pronounced. A gentle touch might feel ticklish or even irritating, sparking a sudden need to pull away. Alternatively, a woman might require firmer pressure or more pronounced stimulation to fully enjoy the experience. Add to this the mental chatter of ADHD—racing thoughts, worries about tomorrow's schedule, or a hyperfocus on a small detail in the room—and it's easy to see how maintaining a seamless flow of physical connection can be challenging.

Overstimulation can also arise from multiple simultaneous sensory inputs: the warmth of your partner's body, the background music, the flicker of candlelight, the pressure of a weighted blanket, and any emotional undertones. If the combined effect is too intense, it can lead to irritability, anxiety, or a sudden shutdown. Conversely, **understimulation** can cause restlessness or distractibility—leading a woman to mentally wander away from the intimate moment in search of more engaging sensations or thoughts.

Overstimulation vs. Understimulation

To better navigate intimacy, it helps to identify whether you're prone to overstimulation or understimulation—or a mix of both. Here's a brief breakdown:

- **Overstimulation**

  1. Symptoms: Irritability, anxiety, feeling overwhelmed, a strong urge to push your partner away or to turn off certain sensory inputs (lights, music).
  2. Possible Triggers: Too many noises, strong scents (e.g., perfumes, scented candles), multiple forms of touch occurring at once, emotional stress.
  3. Coping Strategies: Lowering the lights, reducing background noise, using unscented or lightly scented products, focusing on slow, deliberate touch.

- **Understimulation**

  1. Symptoms: Boredom, distractibility, difficulty maintaining focus on the present moment, seeking more intensity or novelty.
  2. Possible Triggers: Long, slow routines with little variation, subdued or repetitive touch, a lack of mental or sensory engagement.

3. Coping Strategies: Introducing variety in touch (alternating pressures or temperatures), incorporating more dynamic activities (e.g., playful teasing), or using mental imagery and role-play to pique interest.

It's not uncommon for women with ADHD to swing between these states even during a single intimate encounter. What starts as pleasurable and exciting can quickly become too much. Conversely, a session that feels soothing at first might suddenly become uninteresting, prompting the mind to wander. Recognizing these shifts—and communicating them—is a vital step toward deeper connection and sustained pleasure.

Emotional Intimacy and ADHD

Sensory experiences only tell part of the story. Emotional intimacy—the sense of closeness, safety, and mutual understanding between partners—is equally crucial for satisfying sex. Yet, ADHD can complicate emotional bonding. Consider a woman whose ADHD fosters **rejection sensitivity**, a heightened fear of being rejected or criticized. A single offhand comment from her partner can feel like a personal slight, triggering intense hurt or anger. If she internalizes this reaction without expressing it, resentments can build, creating distance rather than closeness.

Moreover, **emotional dysregulation** can lead to rapid mood swings during conflict. A minor disagreement about household chores might escalate into tears or shouting, leaving partners feeling whiplashed by the intensity. If unresolved, these emotional flare-ups can erode trust and safety—bedrocks of a healthy intimate relationship. When repeated conflicts go unchecked, it becomes harder to relax enough to enjoy sex or to feel confident sharing one's body and vulnerabilities.

On the flip side, ADHD can also enhance emotional intimacy when well-managed. The same heightened sensitivity can translate to a profound capacity for empathy or understanding. A woman might sense her partner's emotional cues acutely, responding with warmth or spontaneous acts of affection. Additionally, the **hyperfocus** phenomenon can transform early relationship stages into periods of intense bonding, where each partner feels uniquely seen and valued.

Practical Techniques for Sensory Regulation

Managing the ebbs and flows of sensory input is key to creating a comfortable environment for intimacy. Here are some strategies:

- **Set the Stage**
- **Lighting**: Opt for dimmable lights or soft lamps. Harsh overhead lighting can be jarring.
- **Sound**: If music helps, choose calming or familiar playlists. If silence is more soothing, ensure you can minimize background noise. White noise machines or earplugs can be a lifesaver for those sensitive to ambient sounds.
- **Temperature**: Keep blankets, fans, or temperature controls handy. The slightest feeling of being too hot or too cold can derail focus and comfort.

- **Sensory-Friendly Tools**

- **Weighted Blankets**: Many people with ADHD find that gentle pressure alleviates anxiety. A weighted blanket can provide a calming effect during cuddling or foreplay.
- **Textured Items**: For those who crave novelty, experiment with different textures—silk, velvet, faux fur—on bedding or lingerie to engage the senses in a controlled, pleasurable way.
- **Scent Management**: If strong scents overwhelm you, consider unscented skincare products or lightly scented essential oils that you know you enjoy.

- **Mindful Touch**
- **Slow Progression**: Start with soft, light touches and gradually increase pressure. This helps you gauge your comfort level.
- **Verbal Cues**: Develop a language with your partner for "I need a pause," "That feels really good," or "Could you try something different?" Clear, concise communication prevents misunderstandings or lingering discomfort.
- **Temperature Play**: For under-stimulated minds, alternating between warm and cool sensations—such as using a warmed massage oil followed by a cool breeze from a fan—can sustain engagement and curiosity.

- **Sensory Check-Ins**
- Every few minutes, pause to ask yourself: "How does my body feel right now?" or "Is there anything I need to

adjust?" Encourage your partner to do the same, fostering a collaborative approach to ensuring mutual comfort.

Building Emotional Connection

Navigating sensory needs is crucial, but so is the emotional landscape. Consider these approaches for fostering deeper connection:

- **Open, Non-Judgmental Dialogue**
- Make regular check-ins a part of your relationship, not just your intimate moments. Discuss any ADHD-related stressors—like a tough work week or trouble sleeping—that might influence your mood or interest in sex.
- Practice active listening by giving your partner your full attention, paraphrasing what they say, and offering empathy. This can soothe concerns about feeling unheard or misunderstood.

- **Plan Together**
- For many women with ADHD, spontaneity has its charm but can also be stressful if life is already chaotic. Sometimes, scheduling an intimate evening can be liberating—removing uncertainty and allowing time to mentally prepare and optimize the environment.
- Invite your partner into the planning process, discussing lighting preferences, potential new activities to explore, or ways to handle interruptions (like phones or pets).

- **Use Creative Communication Tools**
- If verbalizing feelings in the heat of the moment is hard, try journaling together or leaving voice notes about what worked and what didn't in a previous intimate encounter. ADHD brains often process thoughts more effectively in writing or with some "thinking space" rather than on the spot.

- **Seek Support When Needed**
- Couples therapy or sex therapy with a professional experienced in ADHD can provide a structured environment for honest conversations. Such a setting helps both partners learn coping strategies and fosters mutual understanding.

Navigating Conflicts and Sensory Overload

Disagreements, misunderstandings, and conflicts happen in every relationship. For couples where at least one partner has ADHD, these challenges can become magnified when sensory sensitivities or emotional dysregulation come into play. One small spark—a comment about the messy kitchen—can escalate if one or both partners are already overstimulated or stressed.

- **De-Escalation Strategy**: Agree beforehand on a signal or keyword that indicates either partner needs a break. It might be as simple as saying, "Time out." During that break, each person can practice grounding techniques—deep breathing, stepping outside for fresh air, or using a stress ball.
- **Return to Discussion**: Once emotions have calmed, revisit

the disagreement with a focus on problem-solving rather than blame. Encourage "I statements" to express how you feel without accusing your partner.
- **After-Conflict Intimacy**: Reconnecting physically after a conflict can be healing. Still, be mindful of any lingering tension or sensory overload. Sometimes, gentle cuddling or a shared bath might be more beneficial than jumping straight into sexual activity.

Embracing Novelty and Play

While managing overstimulation is critical, many women with ADHD also thrive on novelty and playfulness. The ADHD mind can grow bored with routine quickly, and this extends to the bedroom. Introducing **new elements**—like role-play scenarios, sensory toys, or even changing the ambiance—can keep intimacy fresh. This approach isn't about constantly chasing bigger thrills; rather, it's about embracing a spirit of curiosity and adaptability.

- **Small Twists**: If you always use the bedroom, try a different location in your home or vary the time of day you connect intimately.
- **Playful Games**: Consider board games with a romantic or sexy twist, or create a "sensory menu" for each other, listing preferred types of touch, scents, and music, then take turns choosing an item from the menu.
- **Shared Exploration**: For some, reading a book about sensuality or taking an online workshop together can spark fresh ideas. This sense of shared discovery can deepen emotional intimacy.

Communication as the Cornerstone

Ultimately, clear and compassionate communication lies at the heart of managing both sensory overload and emotional connection. When a woman with ADHD feels safe expressing her needs—without fear of judgment or rejection—she's better able to navigate the complexities of her condition and how it intersects with intimacy. By the same token, partners who feel heard and included in the process are more likely to respond with empathy and patience.

For many couples, the process of establishing this communication framework is ongoing. ADHD is dynamic, and needs may shift with hormonal changes, life stressors, or treatment adjustments. Viewing intimacy as a **collaborative journey** rather than a set destination can alleviate pressure and foster a spirit of joint exploration.

Moving Forward

Intimacy and connection for women with ADHD can be a winding path marked by spikes of intense pleasure, abrupt shifts in focus, emotional surges, and sometimes uncomfortable sensory overload. But this path also offers unique opportunities for creativity, empathy, and growth. By acknowledging the role ADHD plays in your sensory and emotional world, you can set more realistic expectations, communicate openly, and design intimate experiences that honor your mind and body.

As you integrate these strategies, remember that you don't need to change who you are to enjoy fulfilling intimacy. Rather, you're learning to work with the rhythms of your ADHD, shaping environments and routines that enhance comfort and connection. Small adjustments—like turning off certain lights, creating a consistent bedtime ritual, or checking in with a partner about sensory needs—can make a profound difference in how you experience and share pleasure.

In our next chapter, we'll delve into **Communication in Relationships**, taking a closer look at the practical frameworks and tools that help women with ADHD express their desires, boundaries, and concerns. We'll also explore common pitfalls—like impulsive outbursts or forgetfulness—and offer concrete methods to navigate them gracefully.

For now, take a moment to reflect on your own experiences with sensory input. Have you noticed times when certain smells or sounds became overwhelming during intimate moments? Do you recognize patterns of seeking out novelty or struggling to maintain focus? Identifying these personal patterns is the first step toward cultivating deeper self-awareness. From there, you can craft the intimate life you truly want—one that accommodates the intricacies of ADHD while celebrating its potential for creativity, spontaneity, and richly felt emotion.

6

Communication in Relationships

The Crucial Role of Communication

The bedrock of any healthy relationship—romantic, sexual, or otherwise—is communication. Yet, for many women with ADHD, talking openly about needs, desires, and challenges can feel daunting. Maybe there's a fear of judgment or a concern about sounding "too much." Or perhaps the chaos of everyday life leaves little mental bandwidth to express complex emotions. Whatever the reason, when communication falters, misunderstandings grow. And once misunderstandings accumulate, they can cast a shadow on intimacy, trust, and emotional safety.

In this chapter, we'll explore how ADHD influences communication patterns, offering both pitfalls and potential strengths. We'll also discuss practical frameworks and strategies to help you and your partner(s) navigate conversations about everything from household logistics to sexual preferences. By understanding common ADHD-related hurdles—like impulsive speech or forgetfulness—you can actively work to bridge gaps and create an environment of mutual respect.

How ADHD Shapes Communication

Living with ADHD often means juggling a swirl of thoughts, feelings, and external stimuli at any given moment. This can manifest in several ways that directly impact communication:

- **Impulsivity**
- Speaking before fully thinking through what you want to say is a common ADHD trait. While impulsivity can sometimes lead to spontaneous expressions of love or creativity, it can also result in blurting out hurtful comments, interrupting someone mid-sentence, or steering a conversation off track.

- **Distractibility**
- Sustaining focus in a conversation—especially if it's lengthy or emotionally charged—may be challenging. You might zone out, miss crucial details, or jump topics without warning. This can leave partners feeling unheard or confused.

- **Emotional Reactivity**
- Many women with ADHD experience heightened emotional responses. A small disagreement can trigger strong reactions—tears, anger, or sudden withdrawal—making it difficult to maintain a calm, constructive tone during conflict resolution.

- **Forgetfulness**
- Even the most attentive listener can forget details days or even hours after a conversation, especially when under stress. Repeatedly forgetting what was discussed can breed frustration and misunderstanding in relationships.

- **Hyperfocus**
- On the flip side, ADHD can enable periods of intense focus or obsession with a topic—such as a new relationship. During these phases, you might communicate tirelessly with a partner about your shared interests. Later, when hyperfocus shifts, you may not sustain the same level of engagement, which can confuse your partner.

Recognizing these patterns is the first step to steering your communication toward greater clarity and empathy. While ADHD can pose challenges, it also brings strengths like creativity, passion, and a capacity for deep empathy—when channeled effectively.

Identifying Common Communication Pitfalls

1. Interrupting or Talking Over

Women with ADHD may unintentionally interrupt others due to impulsivity or fear of forgetting a thought. This habit, however unintentional, can make a partner feel disrespected or overshadowed.

Solution: Practice **active listening**—focus on what your partner is saying, repeat or paraphrase to confirm understanding, and only then share your viewpoint. If you find it difficult to hold onto a thought, jot down a quick keyword on paper or your phone so you can return to it after your partner finishes speaking.

2. Avoiding Conflict

Because conflict can trigger intense emotions, some women with ADHD become adept at "people-pleasing" or sidestepping difficult topics entirely. Over time, unvoiced grievances accumulate, leading to resentment or sudden emotional blowouts.

Solution: Use structured techniques like the **"Sandwich Method,"** where you open with a positive observation, address the concern in a factual, non-accusatory tone, and close with an appreciation or reassurance. This structure can ease anxiety around conflict.

3. Rambling or Going Off-Tangent

ADHD minds often leap from one idea to another in rapid succession, making conversations meandering or hard to follow. Partners may feel lost or impatient.

Solution: **Set a goal** for each conversation—know the main point you want to address. If you notice yourself veering off, pause and ask, "Does this relate to what we're discussing?" If not, note it down for later.

4. Mixed Messages

Due to emotional reactivity, your verbal expression might clash with your nonverbal signals. You say you're "fine," but your crossed arms and shaky voice suggest otherwise. Inconsistencies can create confusion and mistrust.

Solution: Cultivate self-awareness by checking in with your body language and tone. If you sense incongruence, try statements like, "I'm saying I'm okay, but I realize I sound upset. Let me clarify how I really feel."

Conversation Frameworks for ADHD Minds

Having a guiding structure can transform how you approach challenging conversations. Here are a few frameworks that can be particularly useful:

- **HALT: Hungry, Angry, Lonely, Tired**
- Before diving into a sensitive topic, ask yourself: "Am I hungry, angry, lonely, or tired right now?" If yes, address those needs—grab a snack, cool down, connect with a friend, or rest—before initiating the conversation. Doing so reduces the likelihood of emotional outbursts.

- **The Three-Part Message**
- **Observation**: "When X happens..." (state the situation without blame)
- **Feeling**: "I feel..." (describe your emotion)
- **Need/Request**: "I need/prefer/would like..." (be specific about the desired outcome or change)
- Example: "When we make dinner plans and then you cancel at the last minute, I feel disappointed and frustrated. I need more advance notice if you have to change our plans."
- This structure helps keep the focus on the issue, not the person, and guides you toward a potential solution.

- **Check-Backs**
- After a conversation, especially one that's emotionally

intense, schedule a follow-up discussion or use a quick text check-in: "How are we both feeling about what we discussed earlier?" This ensures nothing crucial was forgotten or misunderstood, a common occurrence with ADHD.

- **Time-Limited Talks**
- For lengthy or potentially heated subjects, set a timer for each person to speak uninterrupted for a few minutes. This prevents interruptions and ensures each person gets a turn. After each session, summarize key points before resetting the timer.

The Role of Boundaries

Boundaries aren't just about saying "no" or limiting behaviors; they're also about clarifying **what you need** to feel safe and respected in a relationship. Women with ADHD might struggle with boundaries due to fear of rejection or conflict. However, establishing and honoring personal limits is essential for healthy communication.

- **Emotional Boundaries**: Let partners know if certain topics are off-limits when you're already feeling overwhelmed. For example, "I'm not ready to discuss finances tonight because I'm exhausted. Can we set a time tomorrow?"
- **Physical Boundaries**: This includes comfort with touch, personal space, and environment. If you're sensory-sensitive, communicate that you need a quiet space or minimal distractions to discuss important matters.

- **Time Boundaries**: ADHD can sabotage schedules, but also, some discussions genuinely require an agreed-upon time slot. Plan your conversations when you're both relatively calm and free from urgent tasks.

Conflict Resolution & Repair

No relationship is conflict-free, especially when ADHD's emotional reactivity and distractibility enter the picture. The key is not to avoid conflict but to manage it in a way that leads to growth rather than emotional distance.

- **Cooling-Off Period**
- If a dispute escalates quickly, it's often better to pause before harsh words or impulsive actions cause damage. Clearly state that you need a **cooling-off period**: "I'm feeling overwhelmed right now. Can we revisit this in 20 minutes?"
- During the break, engage in a soothing or grounding activity—listen to music, take a short walk, practice deep breathing. When you reconvene, you'll likely be calmer and more receptive.

- **Apologies That Count**
- A meaningful apology acknowledges the specific hurt caused, not just the act. Rather than "I'm sorry you feel that way," try "I'm sorry I raised my voice earlier. I realize it was hurtful, and I'll try to stay calmer next time." This validates your partner's feelings and demonstrates willingness to change.

- **Solution-Focused Dialogue**
- Once emotions have cooled, shift from blaming to problem-solving. Questions like, "How can we avoid this scenario in the future?" or "What do we both need to feel secure?" keep the conversation collaborative.

- **Seeking Professional Help**
- If conflicts become repetitive or deeply entrenched, a couples therapist—particularly one knowledgeable about ADHD—can provide tools and mediate discussions. Therapeutic settings offer a safe space to practice new communication skills and address underlying resentment or misunderstanding.

Incorporating Technology and Tools

Technology, often seen as a distraction, can be reframed as an ally for ADHD-friendly communication. Apps and tools can help organize thoughts, remember key points, and facilitate respectful conversations:

- **Shared Calendars**: Use Google Calendar or another platform to schedule important discussions or events. Set reminders 24 hours ahead so you both prepare mentally.
- **Note-Sharing Apps**: Platforms like Evernote, OneNote, or Apple Notes allow real-time collaboration. During a talk, you can note agreements or action items. This minimizes the risk of forgetting critical details.
- **Messaging Guidelines**: If texting or messaging apps feel

overwhelming, establish agreed-upon boundaries: for instance, no heavy topics via text, or a "three messages in a row" limit before pausing for a response.
- **Voice Memos**: If you struggle to write down or remember conversation points, record a voice memo to revisit later. Just ensure your partner is comfortable with the recording process and respects any privacy concerns.

The Importance of Listening

Communication isn't just about expressing your side; it's equally about truly **hearing** the other person. Women with ADHD might find active listening a challenge due to distractibility, but with mindful effort, it can become a powerful skill:

- **Minimize Distractions**: Close laptops, silence phones, and turn off the TV. Visual clutter can also be distracting, so choose a calm environment if possible.
- **Reflective Listening**: After your partner speaks, summarize what you heard. "It sounds like you're upset about me forgetting our date. You felt ignored and unimportant." This helps confirm you've grasped the essence of their feelings.
- **Validate Emotions**: You don't have to agree with every detail to acknowledge your partner's emotional experience. Phrases like, "I can see why you'd feel that way," build trust and empathy.
- **Ask Clarifying Questions**: If something is unclear or you sense a detail might have been lost, politely ask, "Could you elaborate on that?" or "Do you mean X or Y?"

Balancing Independence and Collaboration

One unique dynamic in many ADHD relationships is the tension between independence and dependence. Some partners may become caretakers, taking on tasks that feel overwhelming to the ADHD partner. This can foster resentment if not managed. Conversely, the ADHD partner may feel infantilized or overly controlled.

Clear communication about responsibilities helps maintain a healthier balance. If you struggle with certain tasks—like paying bills on time or remembering important appointments—acknowledge it. Collaborate on solutions: maybe an automated app handles bill payments, or you set calendar reminders for deadlines. By treating these logistical challenges as team problems rather than personal failings, you alleviate blame and create an environment of mutual support.

When Communication Becomes Overwhelming

Even with these tools, there will be days when communication feels like an uphill battle. ADHD symptoms can fluctuate with hormonal changes, stress, or exhaustion. During particularly tough periods:

- **Communicate About the Difficulty**: If you're having a high-symptom day, let your partner know. This transparency prevents misunderstandings about short tempers or seemingly distracted behavior.
- **Prioritize Self-Care**: Sometimes, the best strategy is to address your own needs first—whether that's taking a nap, doing a short meditation, or engaging in a calming hobby.

Clearer communication often follows from a calmer mental state.
- **Seek External Support**: Lean on your therapist, a support group, or close friends who understand your ADHD challenges. Processing feelings with someone else can release pressure before you bring the topic to your partner.

Looking Ahead

Effective communication requires ongoing effort, especially when ADHD's impulsivity, distractibility, and emotional reactivity come into play. But by embracing proactive strategies—such as conversation frameworks, mindful listening, and technology tools—you can build a relationship dynamic where both partners feel heard, validated, and respected.

This foundation of healthy communication profoundly impacts sexual and emotional intimacy. When you and your partner can openly share needs, frustrations, and desires, it paves the way for deeper trust, less conflict, and a more authentic connection. In the next chapter, we'll explore a topic that can further complicate or enrich relationships: **ADHD, Trauma, and Sexuality**. We'll examine how past traumatic experiences intersect with ADHD traits and offer pathways to healing and reclaiming sexual agency.

For now, remember that communication is an evolving skill— a dance between speaking and listening, offering and receiving. There will be missteps, especially on stressful days. But with each honest conversation and each willingness to adapt, you build a stronger bond. Embrace the fact that your ADHD brain can bring warmth, empathy, and creativity to communication, so long as you also respect your limits and harness the tools that keep conversations on track. Step by step, you can shape a relational world where all parties feel truly seen and understood.

7

ADHD, Trauma, and Sexuality

The Overlapping Landscape of Trauma and ADHD

Trauma can linger in the body and mind, shaping how you perceive, respond to, and engage with the world. For women with ADHD, the presence of past or ongoing trauma can compound an already complex interplay of emotional regulation, sensory processing, and identity formation. While trauma can arise from a variety of experiences—ranging from childhood abuse to bullying, from toxic relationships to sexual assault—what links them is their power to disrupt a person's sense of safety and control.

ADHD often involves heightened sensitivity and reactivity, making it easier for traumatic events or environments to profoundly affect self-esteem, relationships, and sexual well-being. If you've experienced trauma, you may find that ADHD symptoms (like distractibility, impulsivity, or emotional volatility) amplify distressing memories or triggers. Conversely, trauma can magnify ADHD symptoms, leading to deeper cycles of shame, guilt, or isolation. In this chapter, we'll explore how trauma manifests for women with ADHD, how it intersects with sexuality, and what steps can support healing and reclaiming sexual autonomy.

Recognizing Trauma's Impact on Sexuality

Women with trauma histories often struggle to feel safe in their bodies—a foundation crucial for experiencing pleasure and intimacy. Even if the trauma itself wasn't explicitly sexual, it can still disrupt trust in oneself or in potential partners. For example, if you grew up in a chaotic household where emotional outbursts were frequent, you might have learned to constantly anticipate danger. This hypervigilance can persist in adulthood, making it hard to relax during intimate moments.

When ADHD is part of the picture, **hypervigilance** may be accompanied by distractibility. Perhaps you desperately want to stay present with a partner, but your mind won't stop scanning the environment for potential threats—or it drifts into flashbacks of a past hurt. If trauma was sexual in nature, triggers might include certain types of touch, specific words, or even particular scents that recall painful memories. These triggers can spark involuntary physical or emotional responses—shaking, freezing, shutting down—that can feel bewildering or shame-inducing if you don't recognize them as trauma-related.

Moreover, women with ADHD sometimes exhibit **people-pleasing** or conflict-avoidant behaviors, which can make it difficult to express boundaries. A history of trauma may reinforce these tendencies, leading you to endure uncomfortable or unwanted sexual scenarios rather than risk rejection or confrontation. Over time, this pattern can erode your sense of agency, exacerbating feelings of powerlessness that trauma often leaves behind.

Why Women with ADHD May Be More Vulnerable to Trauma

Research suggests that individuals with ADHD can be more vulnerable to experiencing various types of abuse or toxic dynamics. Several factors contribute to this heightened risk:

1. **Impulsivity and Risk-Taking**
2. The impulsivity inherent in ADHD can sometimes lead to putting oneself in risky or unfamiliar situations without fully weighing potential consequences. While risk-taking itself isn't a moral failing, it can increase exposure to predatory individuals or volatile environments.
3. **Difficulty Picking Up Social Cues**
4. Some women with ADHD struggle with reading social cues or spotting red flags in relationships. This challenge can make it harder to detect manipulative or coercive behavior early on.
5. **Desire for Approval or Belonging**
6. Years of feeling "different" or misunderstood can leave a woman with ADHD eager to fit in or maintain a relationship at any cost. An abusive partner might exploit this longing for acceptance, gradually crossing boundaries or escalating harmful behaviors.
7. **Inconsistent Boundaries**
8. ADHD's fluctuations in attention, mood, and energy can result in inconsistent boundary-setting. One day you might be forthright about your limits; the next day, you might feel too overwhelmed to enforce them. This inconsistency

can expose you to additional harm.

Understanding these vulnerabilities is not about assigning blame; rather, it's about recognizing patterns that may elevate the risk of victimization. With awareness, you can build strategies—whether through therapy, support networks, or personal reflection—that bolster resilience and protect your emotional and physical well-being.

Healing from Trauma: An Ongoing Journey

Healing from trauma is rarely a linear process, and it often involves exploring the mind, body, and emotions in a holistic way. If ADHD is part of your everyday reality, you might need to adapt certain healing strategies to account for challenges like distractibility or emotional reactivity. Here are core elements of a trauma recovery framework that many find helpful:

- **Professional Support**
- Therapy is a cornerstone of trauma recovery. Modalities such as **EMDR** (Eye Movement Desensitization and Reprocessing), **Somatic Experiencing**, and **Trauma-Focused Cognitive Behavioral Therapy** can help reprocess traumatic memories and reduce their impact on daily life. It's important to find a therapist experienced with both ADHD and trauma, ensuring they understand the unique interplay of symptoms.

- **Mind-Body Awareness**

- Trauma often disconnects a person from their bodily sensations, while ADHD can pull the mind in a thousand directions. Practices like **mindful meditation**, **yoga**, or **breathwork** foster a gentler, more attuned relationship with your physical self. Even brief, ADHD-friendly exercises—like 60 seconds of focused breathing or progressive muscle relaxation—can help reinstate a sense of grounding.

- **Community and Support Groups**
- Isolation can intensify feelings of shame or hopelessness. Connecting with others who've faced similar challenges—online or in-person support groups—can validate your experiences and reduce stigma. If possible, seek out groups specifically tailored to women with ADHD or trauma survivors, where mutual understanding is already built in.

- **Medication and Holistic Approaches**
- If you take medication for ADHD or co-occurring conditions like anxiety or depression, remember that these prescriptions may affect your emotional baseline. Some women find they need medication adjustments during periods of intense trauma therapy. Additionally, holistic interventions—like maintaining a balanced diet, regular exercise, and adequate sleep—play a critical role in supporting both mental and physical health.

Reclaiming Sexual Autonomy After Trauma

For survivors of sexual trauma, the road to reclaiming pleasure and agency can be especially complex. Many women wrestle with feelings of guilt or confusion about how their bodies responded—or didn't respond—during the traumatic event. Others may avoid sexual contact altogether, fearing retraumatization. These experiences are natural responses to violation and do not reflect a woman's value or desirability.

Here are some paths toward reclaiming a sense of sexual self-ownership:

- **Slow, Deliberate Exploration**
- If returning to partnered intimacy feels overwhelming, begin with solo exploration. Focus on **sensate awareness**: how does it feel to touch your own skin gently or to notice your breath moving through your body? Gradually expand your comfort zone by exploring erogenous zones or experimenting with self-pleasure in a setting where you control all variables.

- **Establish Clear Boundaries**
- If you choose to engage in sexual activity with a partner, **be explicit** about what is or isn't comfortable. Consider using safe words—simple words or short phrases like "red" or "pause"—to indicate when you need to stop or slow down. This structured communication can be especially important if ADHD-related distractibility or confusion arises mid-encounter.

- **Consider Trauma-Sensitive Sex Therapy**
- A licensed sex therapist trained in trauma sensitivity can help you unpack complex emotions around sexual identity, desire, and boundaries. They can also guide partners on how to support your needs without inadvertently triggering flashbacks or discomfort.

- **Celebrate Incremental Progress**
- Healing from trauma doesn't always involve grand leaps. Sometimes, victory is simply noticing that you felt a bit more relaxed during a cuddle session or that you said "no" when something felt off. Each small step in honoring your body's signals is a milestone.

Navigating ADHD Traits During Recovery

While trauma recovery can be intense for anyone, women with ADHD face unique hurdles:

- **Overwhelm from Therapy**: Processing difficult memories can exacerbate ADHD symptoms, making it harder to focus or regulate emotions during and after sessions. It's helpful to schedule therapy at times when you're less stressed or to plan calming activities afterward.
- **Inconsistent Motivation**: You may feel highly motivated to work on recovery one day and avoidant the next. Setting **mini goals** (like practicing a grounding exercise for one minute each day) can make the process more manageable.
- **Hyperfocus on Trauma**: Some women find themselves

obsessively replaying traumatic events, especially when ADHD hyperfocus locks onto distressing memories. Work with a therapist on **mindfulness techniques** or thought-stopping exercises to interrupt ruminations and redirect attention to the present.

Building Emotional Resilience

Trauma can erode one's sense of inner stability, but resilience is a skill that can be nurtured. Here are some approaches aligned with ADHD mindsets:

- **Flexible Coping Strategies**
- What works on one day may not work on another. Keep a list of coping strategies—journaling, art, music, exercise, grounding exercises—so you can choose from a variety when you sense overwhelm creeping in.

- **Positive Self-Talk**
- Combat negative self-beliefs by keeping encouraging notes or mantras visible. Phrases like "I am resilient," "I deserve to feel safe," or "My worth is not defined by trauma" can serve as quick anchors when self-doubt flares up.

- **Mindful Media Consumption**
- Media—TV shows, news, social platforms—can sometimes feature triggers or romanticize trauma. Being selective

about what you watch or read can lessen the emotional toll. If you notice heightened anxiety or flashbacks after certain content, consider filtering it out.

- **Celebrate Strengths**
- ADHD brings unique strengths: creativity, empathy, curiosity, and resilience. Focus on these traits by engaging in activities that let you shine. Whether it's painting, problem-solving at work, or helping a friend, acknowledging your capabilities can counterbalance the weight of trauma memories.

Supporting Each Other in Relationships

If you're in a relationship, your partner(s) can play a supportive role—but only if they understand the interplay between ADHD, trauma, and sexuality. Encourage open conversations:

- **Educate Together**: Share articles or books about trauma and ADHD so your partner can better grasp your experiences. Learning together fosters empathy and reduces blame.
- **Co-Create Boundaries**: Determine what types of touch, language, or environments feel safe. If you need to leave a social event suddenly due to overstimulation, discuss it in advance, so your partner knows how to respond supportively.
- **Practice Shared Coping Techniques**: Engage in grounding exercises together or take a brief walk if you sense a surge of anxiety. Feeling that you're a team can buffer the isolation that trauma survivors often experience.

Looking Forward: Toward Wholeness

Recovering from trauma is not about erasing painful memories or returning to who you were before. It's about integrating the past into a resilient sense of self, regaining control over your body and sexuality, and learning to flourish despite scars. For women with ADHD, this journey can feel like navigating a labyrinth. But within that labyrinth, you can also discover hidden strengths—heightened empathy, creativity in problem-solving, and a fierce protectiveness of your own well-being.

In the next chapter, we'll examine a topic that often intersects with both trauma and ADHD: **Medication, Libido, and Alternatives**. We'll delve into how medications commonly prescribed for ADHD can influence sexual desire, explore possible side effects, and look at holistic approaches that support both mental health and sexual satisfaction.

For now, as you reflect on ADHD, trauma, and sexuality, give yourself credit for the courage it takes to confront these interconnected challenges. Healing is an act of self-empowerment. Whether you're working through therapy, leaning on friends, or slowly rekindling your sexual spark, each step you take is a testament to your resilience. By understanding how trauma impacts your ADHD—and vice versa—you're better equipped to nurture the wholeness and agency you deserve.

8

Medication, Libido, and Alternatives

The Complex Dance of Chemistry

Women with ADHD often walk a tightrope between managing symptoms and preserving quality of life—including sexual health. While medication can substantially improve focus, impulsivity, and emotional regulation, it may also come with unexpected side effects, such as altered libido or difficulties with sexual performance. On the flip side, some women report that once their ADHD symptoms are under control, they can finally relax enough to enjoy and even enhance their sexual experiences. Clearly, there is no one-size-fits-all story when it comes to ADHD medications and sexuality.

In this chapter, we'll delve into the potential impact of various ADHD treatments—both pharmaceutical and non-pharmaceutical—on sex drive, arousal, and overall satisfaction. We'll also explore strategies to help you work with your healthcare provider to find a balance that supports not only symptom management but also your sexual well-being.

Common Medications for ADHD

The most frequently prescribed medications for ADHD fall into two main categories: **stimulants** and **non-stimulants**.

- **Stimulants**
- **Examples**: Methylphenidate (Ritalin, Concerta), amphetamine salts (Adderall), dexmethylphenidate (Focalin).
- **How They Work**: Stimulants primarily increase the availability of dopamine and norepinephrine in the brain, improving focus and reducing hyperactivity and impulsivity.
- **Potential Sexual Side Effects**: Some women report decreased libido or difficulty achieving orgasm, while others experience enhanced focus that improves arousal and satisfaction.

- **Non-Stimulants**
- **Examples**: Atomoxetine (Strattera), guanfacine (Intuniv), clonidine (Kapvay).
- **How They Work**: Non-stimulants regulate neurotransmitters more gradually and are often chosen for individuals who don't tolerate stimulants well or have certain health conditions.
- **Potential Sexual Side Effects**: These can vary widely. Atomoxetine, for instance, might cause reduced libido in some cases, but others experience no change or even improved functioning due to reduced ADHD-related anxiety.

Some women are also prescribed **antidepressants** (such as SSRIs or SNRIs) to manage co-occurring conditions like anxiety or depression. These medications can also affect sexual desire or function—either dampening libido, delaying orgasm, or occasionally enhancing mood enough to increase interest in intimacy.

How Medication Can Affect Libido

There's no universal rule governing how each medication will influence sex drive—our brains and bodies respond uniquely to chemical shifts. However, several common patterns emerge:

- **Increased Focus, Decreased Spontaneity**
- For some women, stimulants sharpen concentration and help regulate emotions, indirectly boosting sexual desire because they're less anxious or scatterbrained. Yet, the same medication can sometimes reduce that "spark" of impulsivity or spontaneity, altering the individual's sense of sexual excitement.

- **Heightened Emotional Control**
- By smoothing out intense highs and lows, ADHD medications might make women feel more stable. Emotional stability can foster deeper intimacy, but occasionally, women might miss the "edge" they associated with high arousal states. This can manifest as a perceived decrease in passion, even though emotional wellness may be improved overall.

- **Physical Side Effects**
- Some stimulants can cause **dry mouth**, **insomnia**, or **increased heart rate**—factors that indirectly dampen libido or comfort. Insomnia, for instance, might leave you too exhausted for sex.
- In contrast, certain non-stimulants (like guanfacine) might induce sedation, which can be helpful for anxiety but detrimental to sexual energy if it leads to excessive sleepiness.

- **Psychological Shifts**
- Medication can also influence self-esteem. Feeling more "in control" of ADHD symptoms may boost confidence, directly enhancing one's sense of sexual desirability. On the other hand, if side effects (like weight fluctuation or jitteriness) create body-image concerns, libido could take a hit.

Conversations with Your Healthcare Provider

Open communication with your healthcare provider is crucial when medication changes or side effects impact your sexual life. Too often, women feel embarrassed bringing up sexual concerns during routine check-ups, yet doctors can only help if they know what's happening.

- **Be Specific**: Instead of saying, "My sex life is off," describe tangible changes: "I'm having trouble reaching orgasm since starting this medication," or "My interest in sex dropped dramatically in the past month."
- **Track Patterns**: If possible, keep a brief journal noting

dosage, timing, mood, and sexual experiences or desires. Identifying patterns—like reduced libido in the evening if you took medication late in the day—can guide adjustments.
- **Explore Dosage Adjustments**: Sometimes, **lowering the dose** or switching to an **extended-release formula** can mitigate side effects without sacrificing symptom control.
- **Discuss Multi-Medication Regimens**: If you're on additional prescriptions (e.g., birth control, antidepressants, anxiety meds), inquire about **drug interactions** that may compound sexual side effects.

A collaborative approach is ideal: you're the expert on your body; your provider has medical expertise. Working together, you can experiment with strategies to optimize both mental health and sexual fulfillment.

Beyond Medication: Holistic and Alternative Approaches

Medications aren't the only route to managing ADHD symptoms or boosting sexual well-being. Many women find that combining pharmacological treatments with holistic approaches yields the best overall results—especially if they're mindful about potential interactions.

- **Nutrition and Supplements**
- **Omega-3 Fatty Acids**: Found in fish oil, flaxseeds, and walnuts, omega-3s have been linked to improved brain health and mood regulation. Some studies suggest they may mildly help ADHD symptoms, although more research is needed.
- **Iron, Zinc, and Magnesium**: Deficiencies in these miner-

als can exacerbate ADHD symptoms, including fatigue or irritability. Checking levels through a simple blood test and supplementing if needed may support cognitive function and, indirectly, sexual energy.
- **Herbal Teas and Extracts**: Options like ginseng or ashwagandha might offer stress relief, though empirical evidence for ADHD-specific benefits is mixed. Always consult a healthcare professional before starting new supplements, especially if you're on medication.

- **Exercise and Movement**
- **Cardiovascular Activities**: Aerobic exercise (running, dancing, cycling) can boost dopamine levels, improving focus and reducing restlessness. Over time, enhanced mood and energy can translate into heightened sexual interest.
- **Mind-Body Exercises**: Yoga, Pilates, or gentle stretching can help with **body awareness** and stress relief, reducing the distractibility or tension that often undermines sexual enjoyment.
- **Novelty and Variety**: Boredom can be a libido-killer for women with ADHD. Switching up your workout routine—perhaps trying a new dance class—can maintain mental engagement and overall vitality.

- **Therapy and Counseling**
- **Cognitive Behavioral Therapy (CBT)**: Helps reframe negative thought patterns about self-worth or body image,

which can be tied to low libido.
- **Mindfulness-Based Techniques**: Learning to stay present can improve both ADHD symptoms and sexual pleasure, as it trains you to savor sensations without judgment or drift.
- **Sex Therapy**: A specialized approach that focuses on issues like desire discrepancy, communication around sexual preferences, and navigating medication side effects. Some sex therapists also have experience with ADHD-specific challenges.

- **Lifestyle Adjustments**
- **Sleep Hygiene**: Poor sleep worsens ADHD symptoms and can tank libido. Set consistent bedtimes, reduce screen time before bed, and tailor your environment (dark curtains, a comfy mattress) to encourage restful sleep.
- **Reducing Stimulants**: While stimulants are a mainstay of ADHD treatment, external stimulants like caffeine or nicotine can compound jitteriness or anxiety. Moderating caffeine intake, particularly in the afternoon or evening, can improve nighttime relaxation and sexual readiness.
- **Stress Management**: Chronic stress floods the body with cortisol, which can reduce sexual desire. Implementing daily stress-busters—like journaling, brief walks in nature, or short guided meditations—makes a notable difference.

Balancing Medication and Natural Strategies

It's not necessarily an either/or proposition: many women thrive on a **combined approach**—a moderate dose of ADHD medication paired with dietary mindfulness, exercise, and therapy. The interplay can be powerful. When medication tempers impulsivity or restlessness, for instance, therapy becomes more fruitful because you can engage more fully in the therapeutic process. Similarly, improved nutrition and consistent exercise might boost your medication's effectiveness, reducing the required dosage.

The key is to **remain flexible**. ADHD can manifest differently over time, and your sexual needs may evolve due to life changes like shifting hormone levels or relationship status. Regularly reassessing your regimen—possibly with periodic check-ins with a psychologist or psychiatrist—helps ensure you're meeting both mental health and sexual satisfaction goals.

Navigating Myths About Natural Remedies

In your search for non-pharmaceutical solutions, you might stumble on a barrage of "miracle cures" for ADHD: from exotic herbs to restrictive diets promising immediate results. While some alternative practices do offer genuine benefits, it's essential to sift through claims critically. Extreme diets or unregulated supplements can be harmful or interact unpredictably with prescribed medication.

Consider these guidelines:

- **Seek Evidence**: Look for peer-reviewed studies, reputable health websites, or trusted professionals when exploring

new remedies.
- **Monitor Changes**: If you adopt a new supplement or diet, track any shifts in mood, focus, or sexual interest. This record can help you determine if a remedy is genuinely helpful or simply coincidental.
- **Beware of All-or-Nothing Claims**: If someone insists that a particular approach will "completely cure" your ADHD and all its effects on your sex life, approach with caution. ADHD is complex, and management rarely comes in a single magic bullet.

Communication with Your Partner About Medication

If you're in a relationship, discussing your medication journey isn't just a personal matter—it can significantly shape your dynamic. Here's how to approach those conversations:

- **Share Information**
- Explain why you're taking medication, what symptoms it aims to address, and possible side effects. This fosters understanding and empathy rather than leaving your partner guessing about mood shifts or sexual changes.

- **Discuss Timing**
- Some women prefer to take stimulants early in the day to minimize evening restlessness or insomnia. If your sexual activity typically occurs at night, mention how medication timing might influence arousal or energy levels.

- **Invite Feedback**
- Encourage your partner to express any observations, both positive and negative. Perhaps they notice you're more emotionally present yet also more fatigued at bedtime. Constructive input can guide adjustments.

- **Set Realistic Expectations**
- Medication is a tool, not an instant fix. Let your partner know you're experimenting to find the right balance. Emphasize that open communication will be crucial during this process.

Knowing When to Switch Gears

Medication decisions—starting, stopping, switching—are best made in collaboration with a qualified healthcare provider. However, there are certain signs that may indicate it's time for a reassessment:

- **Persistent Negative Sexual Side Effects**: If you've tried dosage adjustments or timing changes and still experience a severely diminished libido or chronic difficulty orgasming, it's worth exploring alternatives.
- **Emergence of New Symptoms**: If a new or increased medication triggers panic attacks, severe insomnia, or other problematic symptoms, discuss a possible switch or additional interventions.
- **Life Stage Shifts**: Hormonal changes (pregnancy, menopause), stressors (like a new job), or major life transitions may alter

your medication needs.

Regular follow-ups, whether quarterly or annually, give you a chance to update your healthcare provider on your evolving circumstances and sexual well-being.

Embracing Experimentation and Self-Advocacy

Ultimately, navigating medication, libido, and ADHD is an exercise in self-advocacy. It might feel awkward to voice concerns about sexual function, but your pleasure and quality of life matter. Here are some strategies to bolster your empowerment:

- **Educate Yourself**: The more you understand your medication's mechanism and side-effect profile, the better you can articulate your experience.
- **Trust Your Body**: If you sense something is off—even if it's not a listed side effect—bring it up. Everyone's biochemistry is unique.
- **Persist in Seeking Solutions**: If one provider dismisses your concerns, consider getting a second opinion. You deserve a healthcare team that takes your sexual well-being seriously.
- **Listen to Others But Choose Wisely**: Input from friends or online communities can offer insights, but remember your situation is singular. Adapt advice to your personal context.

Moving Forward

Finding the right balance between medication for ADHD and maintaining a healthy, satisfying sex life is often a process of ongoing calibration. Some women discover a perfect medication match that alleviates symptoms without dulling libido; others rely primarily on alternative methods and reserve medication for high-stress periods. The possibilities are vast, and none are inherently superior—what matters most is aligning with your body's rhythms, emotional needs, and the intimate life you envision.

In the next chapter, **Empowerment and Self-Discovery**, we'll explore tools to build deeper self-awareness and define what sexual autonomy means for you personally. We'll introduce journaling prompts, exercises for identifying desires and boundaries, and routines that can help you manage ADHD while also nurturing your sexual identity.

For now, reflect on your own experience with ADHD treatments and their effects on your libido or sexual comfort. Have you noticed any patterns—improved focus but decreased spontaneity, or vice versa? Have alternative strategies, like adjusting your diet or picking up an exercise routine, made a difference? By bringing an attitude of curiosity rather than judgment to these questions, you're already taking a proactive step in tailoring your ADHD management to honor both your mental health and your sexual well-being.

9

Empowerment and Self-Discovery

Embracing Complexity

By now, you've traveled through a landscape where ADHD, sexuality, relationships, trauma, and self-esteem all intersect. You've read about the ways that attention difficulties, impulsivity, and sensory sensitivities can shape your intimate life—for better and for worse. You've also explored how medication, therapy, and communication strategies can help forge healthier patterns. Amid all these threads lies an essential question: **Who do you want to be, sexually and personally, as a woman with ADHD?** Answering this isn't as simple as picking a label or adopting a strict plan. It's an evolving process of discovery and empowerment, one that invites you to reclaim your body, desires, and unique neurological wiring.

In this chapter, we'll delve into practical exercises, prompts, and strategies designed to deepen self-awareness and foster empowerment. Think of these tools not as homework assignments to be perfected, but as ways to playfully and compassionately explore your inner world. As you embrace the complexity of your ADHD, you may find that the very traits you once saw as obstacles can become pathways to liberation and joy.

The Importance of Self-Definition

Before diving into specific practices, it's crucial to understand why self-definition matters. So often, women with ADHD grow up feeling as though they're perpetually missing a script—struggling to conform to societal expectations while grappling with invisible challenges. When it comes to sexuality, those same societal pressures can multiply. We're told we should be confident, but not too bold; attractive, but not vain; spontaneous, but also organized. And for a woman with ADHD, the frustration might be doubly intense: "Why do I always feel out of sync with what's 'normal'?"

Stepping into empowerment means **writing your own script**—identifying what truly matters to you, what brings you pleasure, and how you wish to express yourself, both in and out of the bedroom. When you shape your identity on your own terms, you begin to break free from the loop of guilt, shame, or perceived inadequacy.

Self-Reflection: Guided Journaling Prompts

Journaling can offer a safe, flexible container for your thoughts and feelings. Below are a few prompts to spark self-reflection around ADHD, sexuality, and personal growth. Feel free to pick and choose the ones that resonate most:

- **Mapping Your Journey**

- *Prompt*: "When I think about my sexual journey thus far, what stand out as pivotal moments—positive or negative?"
- *Purpose*: Identify key experiences that have shaped your current beliefs about sex. You might notice patterns, such as times when ADHD symptoms played a direct role (e.g., impulsive decisions or struggles with sustained attention).

- **Sensory Exploration**
- *Prompt*: "What types of touch, sounds, tastes, or visuals captivate me the most? How do these preferences relate to my ADHD?"
- *Purpose*: Understanding your sensory preferences can illuminate why certain intimate experiences excite you while others feel overwhelming. This insight becomes crucial for communicating needs to a partner.

- **ADHD Superpowers**
- *Prompt*: "Which of my ADHD traits can actually be strengths in my sexual or emotional life?"
- *Purpose*: Shift focus from deficits to assets. Maybe you bring creativity, spontaneity, or heightened empathy into your relationships. Recognizing these strengths bolsters confidence.

- **Boundaries and Desires**

- *Prompt*: "Where do I feel most comfortable setting boundaries in sex and relationships? Are there areas I'd like to be bolder in voicing my needs?"
- *Purpose*: Boundaries aren't just about saying "no"; they're also about defining the experiences you want more of. Clarifying these boundaries can reduce the confusion that sometimes accompanies ADHD decision-making.

- **Future Vision**
- *Prompt*: "If I could shape my ideal sexual identity and lifestyle without constraint, what would it look like? How would I feel, act, and communicate in that future scenario?"
- *Purpose*: Imagining your ideal can be a potent motivator, guiding you toward concrete changes or goals. Even if reality requires compromise, articulating a vision provides direction.

Mindfulness and Meditation for an ADHD Brain

Mindfulness isn't about having a blank mind; it's about noticing thoughts, sensations, and emotions without judgment. For women with ADHD, it can be especially challenging—but also especially rewarding. Mindfulness techniques can help you stay present during sex, reduce anxiety, and heighten pleasure. Here are some ADHD-friendly approaches:

- **Short, Structured Sessions**
- Instead of aiming for a 20-minute silent meditation (which can feel daunting), start with **two- to five-minute intervals**.

Set a timer. Focus on your breath or a guided audio track. If your mind wanders, gently bring it back.

- **Body Scans**
- Conduct a slow mental check-in from head to toe. Notice tension, warmth, tingles, or aches. Don't judge these sensations; simply observe them. This practice can deepen your connection to your body's cues—essential for both everyday well-being and sexual exploration.

- **Sensory Anchors**
- Tap into your ADHD's affinity for sensory input. Light a candle and focus on the flame, or run your fingers over a soft blanket. Let that sensation anchor you in the present moment. When thoughts spiral, return your attention to the texture, smell, or color you're observing.

- **Afterglow Mindfulness**
- Post-intimacy, take a minute to notice how your body feels. Is there a sense of relaxation, excitement, or emotional vulnerability? This simple reflection can help integrate positive experiences, making them easier to recall later.

Exercises for Self-Discovery and Empowerment

Beyond journaling and mindfulness, a variety of creative exercises can spark deeper insight and a sense of personal agency:

- **Pleasure Mapping**
- **Process**: Either alone or with a partner, set aside time to explore different types of touch on your body—light brushing, firm pressure, circular motions, temperature changes. Mentally note areas that feel especially pleasurable or soothing.
- **Outcome**: Develop a personal "pleasure map" of what lights you up (and what doesn't). For ADHD brains that crave novelty, this hands-on approach can be both informative and fun.

- **Vision Boards**
- **Process**: Gather magazines, images, or digital tools like Pinterest. Create a collage reflecting your ideal sense of sexuality—words, images, colors, moods. Embrace spontaneity; ADHD's creative streak can shine here.
- **Outcome**: A visual representation of your desires can serve as inspiration or motivation. Think of it as a tangible reminder that you're actively shaping your sexual identity.

- **Role-Play Scenarios**
- **Process**: Write out or enact short role-play scenes that

represent different facets of your desired sexual persona—confident seductress, playful explorer, nurturing companion. If you're partnered, invite them to participate in a safe, low-pressure way.
- **Outcome**: Role-play can reveal hidden preferences, ease performance anxiety, and allow ADHD's natural creativity to take center stage.

- **Audio or Video Diaries**
- **Process**: If traditional journaling feels too cumbersome, record voice notes or video clips capturing your reflections, hopes, and struggles.
- **Outcome**: Speaking aloud can be cathartic, especially for those who prefer verbal expression. Listening back to your recordings may reveal patterns you hadn't noticed in the moment.

Building Daily Routines to Support Empowerment

Routines can be lifesavers for people with ADHD—particularly when it comes to self-care, stress management, and sustaining the mental clarity needed for empowerment. Even small daily habits can accumulate into significant personal growth:

- **Morning Check-Ins**
- Devote five minutes each morning to assess your emotional state: Are you anxious, excited, or tired? Identify one self-supportive action (e.g., a gratitude list, a cup of herbal tea, a quick walk) to ground yourself before the day unfolds.

- **Body-Positive Affirmations**
- Write a few affirmations about your body and sexuality on sticky notes or in your phone. Examples might be: "My body deserves pleasure," or "I am allowed to explore desire at my own pace." Repeat these during or after brushing your teeth, integrating them into an existing routine.

- **Sensory Breaks**
- Set reminders during the workday to pause for a sensory break—stretch, sip water mindfully, or listen to a favorite song. This helps regulate attention and prevents burnout, leaving more emotional energy for intimate pursuits later.

- **Wind-Down Rituals**
- Implement a short evening routine that signals it's time to transition from "busy day" mode to "rest and connection." This might include dimming the lights, turning off electronics, or playing calming music. When the mind has time to shift gears, it's easier to be present during intimacy or solo self-reflection.

Claiming Your Sexual Autonomy

Empowerment fundamentally involves **autonomy**—the right to make decisions about your body, pleasure, and relationships. For women with ADHD who've battled self-doubt or negative judgments, it can be liberating to realize you have the power to shape your own sexual reality.

- **Assertive Communication**: If you struggle with speaking up for your desires in the bedroom, practice assertive phrases in low-stress contexts. For example, tell a friend, "I'd prefer to try that new restaurant tonight," or ask a coworker, "Could we brainstorm alternatives?" Each moment of assertiveness helps build confidence.
- **Boundary Reinforcement**: Rehearse boundary-setting statements, such as "I'm not comfortable with this," or "I need a break." By normalizing boundary talk in everyday life, you make it easier to apply when sexual or emotional stakes are higher.
- **Community and Role Models**: Seek out blogs, podcasts, or social media accounts run by other women with ADHD who champion body positivity and sexual empowerment. Hearing others' stories can validate your own journey and offer fresh perspectives.

Handling Setbacks and Plateaus

Growth isn't linear—especially with ADHD. One week, you might feel unstoppable, journaling daily and practicing mindful intimacy. The next, life circumstances or an ADHD flare-up can derail your plans. **Plateaus and setbacks** are part of the process, not indications of failure.

When you stumble:

1. **Reassess**: Was your routine too ambitious? Do you need to break your goals into smaller steps? Or is something else, like stress or health issues, taking priority right now?

2. **Practice Self-Compassion**: Treat yourself as you'd treat a good friend who's struggling. Acknowledge disappointment, but resist catastrophizing.
3. **Return to Tools That Work**: Review earlier journal entries or revisit a favorite grounding technique. Familiar coping strategies can serve as emotional and psychological anchors.

Celebrating Milestones

Empowerment thrives on **positive reinforcement**. Celebrating even seemingly small achievements helps sustain motivation, particularly for an ADHD brain that thrives on rewards and novelty:

- **Micro-Celebrations**: Completed a week of mindful check-ins? Treat yourself to a soothing bath or a new eBook.
- **Shared Joy**: If you have a supportive friend or partner, let them know about your milestone. Sometimes, sharing good news amplifies the sense of accomplishment.
- **Visual Reminders**: Keep mementos—like a note in your planner or an object on your desk—that remind you of how far you've come, whether it's a new sexual insight or successfully implementing boundary-setting.

Looking Toward the Final Chapter

As you engage with these exercises and reflections, remember that empowerment isn't about perfection. It's about **presence**—being present to your own desires, quirks, boundaries, and growth, all while acknowledging that ADHD can add layers of complexity. Yet within those layers, many women find newfound self-discovery and pleasure. The challenges you face in focus or emotional regulation can become catalysts for authenticity, creativity, and more nuanced communication in bed and beyond.

In our upcoming, final chapter—**Moving Forward: Embracing Complexity**—we'll synthesize the themes discussed throughout this book. We'll look at long-term strategies for continuing your ADHD and sexual well-being journey, emphasizing community, advocacy, and a vision for ongoing evolution. By now, you've gathered tools, insights, and (hopefully) a sense of affirmation that your experiences are valid. With continued exploration and self-compassion, you can keep shaping a fulfilling intimate life that honors the full richness of who you are.

For the moment, give yourself credit for the willingness to learn, explore, and question. Let each exercise or journaling prompt bring you closer to the core of your desires and strengths. Empowerment isn't a destination but a dynamic, living process—one you're already traveling, step by step, toward a deeper connection with yourself and the kind of sexual and emotional life you truly want.

10

Moving Forward – Embracing Complexity

A Lifelong Journey

You've reached the final chapter of this book, having traveled through the expansive terrain of ADHD and sexuality from a woman's perspective. You've examined how attention-deficit/hyperactivity traits intersect with intimacy, trauma, relationships, and body image. You've delved into practical tools—medication strategies, holistic approaches, communication techniques, sensory-friendly intimacy tips, and empowerment exercises. The question now is: **Where do you go from here?**

It's tempting to see a "last chapter" as an endpoint. In reality, integrating ADHD management with a fulfilling sexual life is an ongoing process. Much like any relationship, your bond with your own body and mind evolves over time. Shifting life circumstances—like career changes, parenting, hormonal fluctuations, or aging—can prompt you to adjust your strategies. What worked wonders last year may need tweaking today.

Rather than viewing this as a sign of failure, you can embrace it as a natural part of growth: an invitation to stay curious, adaptable, and compassionate with yourself.

Celebrating What You've Learned

Before diving into future-oriented strategies, take a moment to celebrate how far you've come. Whether you've tried a single journaling prompt or overhauled your entire approach to intimacy, each step is a milestone.

- **Self-Awareness**: You've gained insight into how ADHD shapes everything from mood and libido to communication styles. Recognizing patterns is the first step in making empowered choices.
- **Tools and Techniques**: From setting boundaries to trying weighted blankets, you now have a repertoire of potential solutions for sensory overload, emotional reactivity, and staying present during sex.
- **Community and Resources**: Perhaps you've reached out to a therapist, joined an ADHD support group, or followed online forums. You've taken concrete actions to reduce isolation and learn from others.
- **Renewed Autonomy**: By reflecting on your desires and boundaries, you're reclaiming agency in your sexual relationships. You have a clearer sense of what you want—and don't want—in your intimate life.

Ongoing Personal Evolution

The concept of evolution is key. ADHD is not a static condition; its impact can ebb and flow with stress levels, hormonal changes, and even significant life events like marriage, career shifts, or grief. Likewise, sexuality is far from a fixed state. Desire can soar or wane, interests can change, and emotional needs can become more nuanced with time.

1. Regular Self-Check-Ins

Periodically pause to assess where you are on your ADHD and sexual well-being journey. Are you feeling fulfilled, curious, or frustrated? Which ADHD symptoms are most pronounced right now, and how might they be influencing your libido or relationship dynamics? These mini "status updates" can guide you in making timely adjustments—whether that's seeking therapy again, changing medication dosage, or experimenting with new ways to ignite desire.

2. Revisiting Past Tools

Don't abandon the strategies that served you well just because circumstances shifted. Instead, adapt them. For example, if scheduling intimate evenings worked wonders at one point but now feels too rigid, try integrating partial spontaneity or new rituals to keep it fresh. Many ADHD-friendly tools, like sensory breaks or mindfulness exercises, can remain valuable mainstays—just reshaped to fit your current reality.

3. Continuing Education

New research on ADHD and sexual health emerges regularly. Stay informed by subscribing to reputable newsletters, following mental health organizations on social media, and reading updated literature. This ongoing learning not only helps you refine your strategies but can also give you a sense of solidarity—knowing there's a growing body of knowledge dedicated to your lived experience.

Fostering Supportive Networks

Maintaining a robust support system is often a game-changer for women with ADHD. When it comes to sexuality, having trusted individuals to confide in—whether friends, therapists, online peers, or romantic partners—can normalize challenges and amplify triumphs.

- **Friends and Peers**
- Look for local or virtual ADHD support groups. Even if they're not specifically about sexuality, these spaces often foster openness about all areas of life. If you need to discuss intimate topics, consider forming a smaller, private subgroup with members who share that focus.
- Seek out friends who are open-minded about discussing sexual well-being. These might be people who've tackled their own challenges and can reciprocate understanding and advice.

- **Healthcare and Therapy**
- Keep an ongoing relationship with a mental health professional who understands ADHD, if possible. This can be especially beneficial during life transitions—like pregnancy, postpartum, or menopause—when hormonal shifts can exacerbate ADHD symptoms and affect libido.

- If you're exploring trauma recovery or nuanced sexual issues, a sex therapist familiar with ADHD can tailor interventions that respect both conditions' complexities.

- **Online Forums and Communities**
- Online spaces—subreddits, Facebook groups, specialized forums—can offer immediate, around-the-clock support. You can pose questions anonymously, share insights, or simply read others' stories. Just remember to balance online advice with professional guidance when necessary.

Advocacy and Raising Awareness

As you gain confidence navigating your own ADHD-sexuality interplay, you might feel compelled to speak up about it more widely. Doing so can benefit not only you but also countless others who feel isolated by stigma or lack of information.

- **Sharing Personal Stories**: If you're comfortable, consider writing blog posts, social media updates, or even articles for mental health and women's publications. Narratives from real individuals can be far more impactful than clinical statistics.
- **Engaging in Community Programs**: Schools, community centers, or mental health nonprofits sometimes welcome guest speakers. By discussing how ADHD affects women's lives—intimacy included—you help shift public perception and improve resources.
- **Lobbying for Better Healthcare**: If you find gaps in the med-

ical system—for instance, a lack of providers who understand female ADHD and sexual well-being—join advocacy groups pushing for improved training and policy changes. Your voice can be a catalyst for more comprehensive care models.

The Power of Continuous Self-Compassion

A central thread running through this entire book is **self-compassion**. ADHD can make daily tasks more complex, and societal messages may amplify feelings of shame. When you add the deeply personal realm of sexuality, the stakes often feel even higher. Self-compassion is what enables you to meet setbacks with understanding rather than self-criticism. It's what allows you to celebrate small victories—like asking for a boundary or trying a new sensory approach in bed—without minimizing those accomplishments.

- **Anchor Phrases**: Develop a short mantra that resonates: "I'm learning at my own pace," or "I can grow through this." Repeat it when you catch yourself spiraling into negative self-talk.
- **Compassionate Journaling**: If journaling resonates with you, use it as a space to practice self-kindness. Write about challenges but also highlight what you did well, no matter how minor.
- **Visual Reminders**: Place gentle reminders of self-compassion in your environment—a sticky note on the bathroom mirror, a phone background, or an alarm labeled "Check in gently."

Reimagining Sexuality with Creativity

Women with ADHD often excel in creativity, which can be a potent asset in the bedroom and beyond. If routine or monotony dulls your sexual desire, **intentionally infuse creativity**:

- **Explore Novelty**: Try new positions, role-plays, or environments if it's safe and consensual. Novel stimuli can engage the ADHD brain, turning intimacy into an exciting adventure rather than a repetitive task.
- **Art and Sexual Expression**: Channel your creativity through painting, photography, or collages that represent your sexual fantasies or emotional landscapes. This form of self-expression can deepen self-awareness and sometimes even spark dialogue with a partner.
- **Collaborate with Partners**: If you're in a relationship, brainstorm ways to keep intimacy fresh. Challenge each other to think of small twists—maybe a "mystery date" night or playful text prompts throughout the day. By co-creating, you maintain a sense of shared discovery.

Addressing Ongoing Mental Health Needs

While this book has focused on ADHD, remember that many women also navigate co-occurring conditions like anxiety, depression, or PTSD. Each of these can significantly affect sexual well-being and relationships. Staying vigilant about your overall mental health—whether through therapy, medication, support groups, or lifestyle strategies—creates a stable foundation for everything else.

- **Periodic Evaluations**: Schedule annual check-ins with a mental health professional or primary care physician, especially if you're using medication. Life stressors can alter how your body responds to medication or therapy.
- **Self-Regulation Tools**: Keep practicing those grounding exercises, relaxation techniques, or scheduling hacks. ADHD management is rarely "one and done"—it's an evolving skill set you refine over time.

Long-Term Vision: Living Authentically

Ultimately, your path forward is about living authentically in every domain. The empowerment and self-discovery exercises you've encountered aren't just about improving sexual pleasure (though that's certainly valuable); they're about honoring your entire being—quirks, desires, challenges, and all.

- **Align with Values**: Reflect on your core values: compassion, growth, adventure, stability, creativity, or connection. How can you ensure your sexual decisions, routines, and relationships align with these values rather than contradict them?
- **Give Yourself Permission**: Permission to change your mind, to evolve, to be uncertain, and to learn from each experience. This openness allows your ADHD to be not a handicap but a compass pointing you toward novel possibilities.
- **Celebrate Your Complexity**: You contain multitudes. You are not just a woman with ADHD, nor just a sexual being, nor just the sum of your roles (mother, partner, professional). Embrace the complexity that makes you uniquely you.

Practical Tips for the Road Ahead

As you integrate the insights from this book, consider these final reminders:

- **Set Realistic Goals**
- Adaptation takes time. Whether it's practicing new communication skills or experimenting with different forms of intimacy, don't overload yourself. Pick one or two focus areas at a time.

- **Track Gradual Progress**
- If you're someone who benefits from structure, keep a monthly or quarterly log of how your ADHD symptoms and sexual satisfaction fluctuate. Look for correlations—are stress levels at work influencing desire? Does a certain supplement or mindfulness routine coincide with better focus?

- **Seek Allies**
- Don't hesitate to ask for help or accountability, whether from a friend, a partner, a therapist, or an online group. Sometimes a simple check-in from someone who understands can spur you to keep going.

- **Stay Adaptable**
- ADHD thrives on novelty and variety. Keep a list of backup strategies for days when your usual approach isn't clicking. Remain open to revisiting earlier chapters or re-trying abandoned techniques under new circumstances.

A Final Word

It's worth repeating: **there is no single "right" way** to be a sexually empowered woman with ADHD. Some days, you might feel unstoppable—engaging in playful intimacy, articulating boundaries with ease. Other days, it might feel like you're back at square one, tripping over forgetfulness or sensory overload. This ebb and flow is part of being human, especially when you have a neurologically diverse mind.

As you close this chapter, remember that you carry forward a wealth of knowledge and practical tools. You know how to communicate your needs, how to manage overstimulation, how to shape a relationship that honors both partners' perspectives, and how to care for your mental and emotional health. Most importantly, you've learned to see yourself through a lens of empathy and self-worth rather than judgment.

The journey continues—through fresh challenges, shifting life phases, and the delightful surprises that come from embracing novelty. When confusion or frustration arises, circle back to the core truths you've discovered in these pages: you are worthy, complex, and capable of creating a sexually and emotionally fulfilling life that celebrates the entirety of who you are.

Thank you for reading, exploring, and allowing this book to be part of your personal growth. May your path forward be rich with self-discovery, empowered decisions, and a deepening sense of connection—to yourself, to those you love, and to the life you're continually crafting.

www.ingramcontent.com/pod-product-compliance
Lightning Source LLC
Chambersburg PA
CBHW071721020426
42333CB00017B/2349